Community Health Systems in the Rural American South

Community Health Systems in the Rural American South

Linking People and Policy

Carole E. Hill

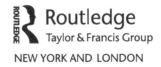

Routledge
Taylor & Francis Group

NEW YORK AND LONDON

First published in 1988 by Westview Press

Published in 2021 by Routledge
605 Third Avenue, New York, NY 10017
2 Park Square, Milton Park, Abingdon, Oxon OX14 4RN

Routledge is an imprint of the Taylor & Francis Group, an informa business

Library of Congress Cataloging-in-Publication Data
Hill, Carole E.
   Community health systems in the rural American South.
   Bibliography: p.
   Includes index.
   1. Rural health services—Southern States. 2. Public health—Southern States. 3. Medical policy—Southern States. 4. Community health services—Southern States.
I. Title.
RA771.6.S63H55   1988   362.1′2′0975   88-214
ISBN 0-8133-7541-X

ISBN 13: 978-0-3670-1439-1 (hbk)
ISBN 13: 978-0-3671-6426-3 (pbk)

Contents

Illustrations

Maps

Preface

A cultural perspective of health care systems can provide health care providers and policymakers with a broader understanding of the issues they face when planning and implementing new health programs in communities. Health care takes place in a community setting while health care policy is developed at an entirely different level in the larger socioeconomic system. While some may think that this is common knowledge, there are few studies that attempt to link the community level systems of health with those of the policy level system and that allow for a comparison of the convergence and divergence of people's health beliefs and behavior with those of policymakers.

In order to help fill the lacunae, I undertook the study of Coberly. My initial interest in medical anthropology in the late 1960s and early 1970s was in "folk medicine." After a rather idealistic attempt to apply my findings to health service delivery by writing and talking about them to health professionals, I decided that if we as anthropologists were to have an impact on health care delivery, we should also analyze the power structure of health and, when possible, create and obtain power positions ourselves in order to effect health policies. The first step was to "study up" and understand the culture of policy and planning. Although this was not a new idea in the discipline, I set out to accomplish this goal by combining a systems approach with a health behavior and beliefs model.

My first step was to study health policy. I was given the opportunity to do so with a post-doctoral fellowship from the Medical Anthropology Program, University of San Francisco. For a year, I studied health planning and policy and began to see the integration between this field and that of anthropology within the framework of rural health. Upon my return to the American South, I designed a research project that would link the policy level of health to that of a rural community. The results of. my efforts are presented in this manuscript.

A major assumption of my analysis is that health care systems are structured and transformed within the larger context of the political, economic, cultural, and social systems in which they exist. Although there are stated health policies on the national and state levels in America, researchers have reported the existence of many health systems beyond biomedicine. People tend to tap into several systems when they are ill. They may consult a doctor and drink teas made from special roots or take vitamin C. The decisions people make are guided by their health knowledge—a part of their cultural model of the world. How they derive this knowledge depends, to a large extent, on the specific social, political, and economic systems in which they live. These systems must be delineated and analyzed on the community level, and on the state and national levels, in order to explain how people intersect and interrelate to the dominant health care system as well as to alternative systems. This type of analysis is crucial for evaluating the effectiveness of health policies designed to transform people's health behavior and beliefs.

For the past few years, I have felt that two inextricably bound concepts in anthropology—culture and structure—hold the key to providing a theoretical perspective that works in the research and applied endeavors of medical anthropology. They are the building blocks of a model that can explain social order on the one hand and social change on the other, in a manner that has practical application. In this book, I attempt to integrate them by taking a modified systems approach that links the macrolevel of the culture and structure (economics and politics) of health policy with the microlevel of the culture and structure (community health beliefs and behavior) of the health system. Too often, medical anthropologists have neglected to go beyond the microlevel (Janzen 1978, Frankenberg 1980, Waitzkin 1978). However, the political and economic structure of a society affects the types of health systems that exist in that society, the resource allocation to support particular health systems, and the degree of integration of the dominant health system with those that exist on the community level. On the other hand, the health realities (cultural models) of the people who participate in the larger systems affect, as well, the changing structure and culture of health within the community; they are themselves directive forces that motivate behavior (D'Andrade 1984). We must keep in mind that although part of people's health reality is determined by the larger system, they affect the effectiveness of health care policies through their decision making. The assumptions of the dominant ideology that underpins the economic and political system are the forces that guide decision making. After all, the health care system is a part of the political, economic, and historical order of a society. As a result, I argue that health care policies and their enforcement depend, to a large extent, on the cultural system of policymakers and their methods of implementation which, in turn, affect the delivery of health services in a community.

In the first five chapters of this book, I present the structure and culture of the "health" in Coberly, a rural community in the American South. I analyze the health problems of the people of Coberly, their illness behavior, their health-seeking behavior, and their beliefs and attitudes about health. As expected, these differ strikingly from the assumptions of policymakers and planners. Beliefs also vary within the community, along the lines of class and ethnicity. On the other hand, I found some similarities, some ideologies shared with the dominant culture and among various groups within the community. Coberly, like all communities, is heterogeneous. It is structured along ethnic and class lines, with the Blacks belonging to the lower socioeconomic levels and the Whites spanning all the class levels. As would be expected, the dominant classes of Whites demonstrate more of a congruence with the ideology of the outside systems than do the lower class groups. Indeed, Chapter 6 demonstrates how the values of a group of white leaders in Coberly intersect with those of the policymakers, providing a systematic linkage that allow for the construction and the meanings that underlie specific rural policies. Overall, I demonstrate that these policies are based on an urban hospital model of medical care that developed with little knowledge of the structure and culture of rural communities.

In Chapter 8, I analyze the convergent and divergent processes that characterize ideological and behavioral aspects of the health and medical systems. I argue that the ways in which policy and people are linked have both theoretical and practical implications for social scientists and for health policymakers and planners.

Any study of a developed or developing nation must take into consideration the concepts of class and ideology, especially if the structural and cultural processes between community and the dominant levels of economic and political structures are to be fully understood. In my analysis, I attempt to integrate the conflict approach to social order and transformation with the symbolic approach. I am assuming that there are always stresses and strains among the health systems. The parts and levels of their structures, however, are not in conflict with one another at all times, nor are the groups on the community level completely dominated ideologically or structurally by the political economy. The linkages that develop between the structures in systems are continually negotiated, bringing about changes on all levels. The systems are always transforming on some level.

Analyzing the culture and structure of health systems provides an opportunity to clarify these processes and to further our knowledge of health behavior within a larger context. For example, the health care system in the United States is dominated by what has been termed a "medical industrial complex," with the scientific biomedical model as the major ideology. Although this model is the basis for most planning and policymaking in service delivery, the beliefs and behavior of the people of Coberly are not limited by it. As I discuss in Chapters 3, 4, and 5, there is a negotiation process between what we term their "traditional system of health" and the dominant medical system. In the past two decades, the people, particularly the lower classes, have had increasing access to clinical medicine. Indeed, it has become pervasive in the lives of many rural dwellers. They consequently have incorporated some of its terminology and values into their overall health behavior and beliefs, while at the same time maintaining their own ideology, thus incorporating into their health ideology the legitimating health ideology of their society. They are aware of the conflicts, but instead of insisting on reordering society, they want equal opportunities and participation in the structuring of their world. Consequently, there are degrees of domination of the less powerful and a variety of interpretations and reinterpretations in the production and reproduction of health knowledge. Increasing access (through intervention), then, expands the culture and structure of the dominant system and links people with divergent health beliefs and behaviors through various processes such as health education, health promotion, and health policies.

In this book I attempt to bridge these systems and levels by describing the health system of a heterogeneous community in the rural South. I use the approach of medical anthropology, a recognized area of study that began after World War II and has grown considerably in the past decade. Medical anthropologists use the entire range of theories and methods within the field of anthropology; they are employed in universities, medical schools, schools of public health, and federal, state, and local agencies. Perhaps because of the diversity of research and applied interests of medical anthropologists, and the diversity of theories and methods in anthropology, medical anthropology has not developed a conceptual framework that goes beyond the polemical arguments for functional, ecological, or ethnomedical analysis or critical theory. Camaroff (1983) calls medical anthropology "a delimited subfield" that leads medical anthropologists to analytical involution or confusion. I believe one reason for confusion about the subfield is the incorporation of the term "medical" into the cultural models we are proposing to study. While we study and work in medical settings, we often use the medical model of western culture to define our conceptual tools. This predicament not only delimits our findings and undermines our objectivity, it also precludes the development of a paradigm for "medical anthropology." It is, nonetheless, a name that has stuck and that identifies a subarea in anthropology that studies folk medicine, health behavior, human adaptation, and medical and cultural change (Lieban 1974). However, medical anthropologists are increasingly practicing their craft outside of the academic setting, finding many of the concepts are useful in applying anthropology to health settings (Hill 1985).

There are many people who supported my research without whom I would have been unable to begin, much less to guide this project to a conclusion. First, the people of Coberly welcomed us into the community and cooperated with us, even though at times some came close to losing patience with all our questions. I appreciate their cooperation. Their names have been changed to fictitious ones in the manuscript as have the names of the towns. Second, the graduate students who worked on the project were dedicated and attended more training and data analysis sessions than they had ever anticipated. They are Pat Thomas, Tom Thrasher, Anne Seagraves, Linda Holbrook, and Frank Jones. I sincerely thank them. Third, I appreciate the cooperation of the health personnel, planners, and policy-makers on the local, state, and national levels. Although some did not agree with the relevance of my research, all were cordial and willing to be interviewed.

The funding for this research came from several research grants from Georgia State University. I appreciate the support of my colleagues and especially my dean, Dr. Clyde Faulkner. The editing of the manuscript was the arduous task of Saralyn Chesnut. I thank her for her perserverance. The task of checking references was admirably carried out by Ivia Cofresi. The typing of the manuscript was done by Steve Fievet and Jean Reed. I appreciate their efforts and support.

Carole E. Hill

References

Cameroff, Jean
    1983   The Defectiveness of Symbols or the Symbols of Defectiveness? On the Cultural Analysis of Medical Systems. Culture, Medicine and Psychiatry 7:3-20.

Frankenberg, Ronald
    1980   Medical Anthropology and Development: A Theoretical Perspective. Social Science and Medicine 14B:197-207.

Hill, Carole E.
    1985   Training Manual in Medical Anthropology. Washington, D.C.: Society for Applied Anthropology/American Anthropological Publication No. 18.

Janzen, John M.
    1978   The Comparative Study of Medical Systems as Changing Social Systems. Social Science and Medicine 12:121-129.

Lieban, Richard
    1974   Medical Anthropology. In Handbook of Social and Cultural Anthropology. John J. Honigman, ed. Pp. 1031-1072. New York, Rand McNally College Publishing Company.

Waitzkin, Howard
    1978   A Marxist View of Medical Care. Annals of Internal Medicine 89:264-278.

1

Culture, Health, and Policy in the Rural South

The issues involved in health care delivery and in assessing its effectiveness and utilization in American society have been topics of intensive research in the social sciences for many years. Currently, one of the most active areas is health services research, which often generates policy on specific health issues such as strategies for client reimbursement, community administration, and distribution of health personnel. A large body of literature produced in the past decade addresses these issues within the contexts of both rural and urban environments. There is also an abundance of literature analyzing the impact of health research on health policy and planning. These bodies of literature, either implicitly or explicitly, raise the crucial issue of the relationship between social science research and public policy.

This study attempts to address that issue by integrating one social science approach—that of anthropology—with that of the policy process. It does so by documenting the implementation of rural primary health care policies in a small community in the American South. In general, a systems model is employed to explore the links between the microlevel (the community) and the macrolevel (the policy process). This integration of the traditional anthropological approach to community studies with that of policy construction and analysis provides a unique opportunity to evaluate the impact our knowledge of health beliefs and behaviors of rural peoples on the effectiveness of current health policies.

In this study, the assumptions and ideologies expressed in rural health policies and by rural health planners about rural populations are compared to the reality of a specific population's culture, including ideas about health,

health behavior and actual needs. Through exploring the differences among various systems of rural policy and the variables that affect these systems, I argue that being able to improve health care services is dependent as much on understanding cultural and social variables in planning and implementing health policies as on medical knowledge. Furthermore, I argue that making medical services available and accessible is only the first step toward providing adequate health care services. The importance of health to a population and its concepts of what health is (cultural models) must be examined as viable variables if the health care system is to solve the overall health problems of a population. This book, then, examines the relationship(s) between rural health policies in the United States and the health beliefs and behaviors of a heterogeneous Southern community.

Health as a Cultural and Social System

Health is something one experiences. It may be evaluated as good or bad depending on one's perception and evaluation of symptoms. This is a relative process that is influenced by a person's beliefs and values. For example, a prevailing assumption among many Americans is that health is a "right" rather than a "privilege" and that every life has an intrinsic worth. More controversial is the debate which asks the question: Who is most responsible for a person's health—the individual or the established health care system? Other questions include who should provide health care, what the content of the medical episode should be or, indeed, what is meant by health or a healthy person. These are all cultural questions. The answers vary and are substantially based on how groups or individuals experience their health within the larger social and cultural systems.

Whatever the answers to these questions for individuals, the ideas and experiences that shape their health behaviors also order their intellectual, social and emotional lives. These ideas and experiences are the "webs of significance" that people have spun, creating meaning in their lives (Geertz 1973). In the American South, ideas related to health and disease, which are rooted in traditional ways of life, now integrate many clinical realities, both traditional and modern. These ideas allow Southerners to make sense of their lives and to cope with anomalies in their everyday affairs (Hill and Mathews 1981). The finite segment of health possibilities thus confers meaning and significance, but it is not arbitrarily chosen; social, economic and political structures become an integral part of the possibilities for meaning. Consequently, meaning results from a dialectical interchange between culture and structure. Political, economic and social structures limit the choices members of a social group may make in order to solve the day-to-day problems of human existence, while the culture of a social group limits the range of meaningful behaviors individuals in the group may choose. Culture both constitutes and is constituted by the structures of a society, in a never-ending process of indeterminacy and change. The dialectic between social structure and culture produces on the one hand a sense of tradition and on the other hand an experience of change (transformation). It is at this juncture that we are able to understand and explain the dynamics of continuity and change in a cultural and social system. The dynamics of the meaning of health to a population, the place of that population in the overall economic and social structure, and the politics that guide the extent and distribution of health services can be explained within this ongoing process.

Indeed, a major determinant of the content and structure of a health care system as well as of its meaning to a populace is the political and economic structure of a society. Any interpretation of the interplay between the health behavior and beliefs of a population (culture) and the health care system (structure) must also consider the economic and political structures of that society. The basis for making decisions that affect health care services (for example power and resource allocation) is a crucial variable in explaining continuity and change in health care systems and their impacts (the constituting factors) on the health cultural system. Indeed, Elling feels that "medical systems change primarily as a result of, or in conjunction with, broad change in national and international political economic orders" (1978:107).

Consequently, health, as a cultural system, must be understood within a political and economic context. Health systems, then, are both cultural systems and social systems. The problem of access to "scientific" medicine, and the meaning of this term to rural populations can illustrate this point. Dow (1976) feels that the poor health of migrants, mountaineers and "dirt farmers" in the South stems from their sense of powerlessness. It is thus the political economy (and the people's place in it) that is, in effect, controlling access to health facilities for both the privileged and the lower classes. Indeed, Dow feels that the successful medical care programs in rural areas are those that are owned and operated by local people. Furthermore, McKeown (1975) has statistically demonstrated that improvements in health in the first half of this century were largely due to economic/environmental factors (better jobs and public health), rather than to medical advances. Thus, health care and disease are not simply medical concerns. They involve the health experience of individual patients, the family, the well-being of the community, and the position and power community members have in the hierarchy of the political and economic structure; they are basically social and cultural phenomena.

Moreover, in the rural South, traditional, non-"scientific" health care beliefs and practices persist. These practices include a wide variety of self-help techniques in the form of home remedies, media medicine, over-the-counter drugs, and the use of traditional healers. Several kinds of folk healers (hoodoo doctors, voodoo doctors, herb doctors, root doctors, and conjurers) heal a variety of illnesses and perform rituals that often solve the contradictions and paradoxes of people's daily existence. By using these remedies and healers, rural Southerners are demonstrating their belief in different concepts of health and illness—concepts that are not acceptable to the mainstream medical establishment. On the other hand, such practices do not preclude the use of scientific medicine. Indeed, rural Southerners integrate both kinds of medicine into a broader belief framework than that of "scientific" concepts, with each representing separate clinical realities.

When rural peoples have equal access to health services, they often integrate the new ideas such services represent into their cultural framework and begin to share some of the health beliefs of the dominant structure and culture. Scientific medicine becomes meaningful and significant. The assumed conflict between traditional medicine and modern scientific medicine is a product of our thinking, not that of rural Southerners (Hill and Mathews 1981). Not surprisingly, then, traditional medicine is often utilized for chronic health problems and scientific medicine for acute health problems. In fact, Southerners' utilization rate of medical services for chronic conditions is 12 percent below that of other regions, although the disability rate is higher than that in other regions (Rogers 1979). Individuals are caught in a dominant system that feeds back on itself through structural policies, and yet they behave and believe in ways that do not necessarily conform to the dominant structure. Gramsci called the dominance of this structure, "cultural hegemony," which creates "an order in which a certain way of life and thought is dominant, in which one concept of reality is diffused throughout society in all its institutions and private manifestations, informing with its spirit all taste, morality, customs, religious and political principal, and all social regulations, particularly in their intellectual and moral connotations" (1971:204). Because rural Southerners are aware of the cultural hegemony of the scientifically based health care system, many are reluctant to discuss their various pathways to health; they just have different illness behavior patterns.

The meaning of health and illness is based on the religious beliefs of rural Southerners. Beliefs about why illnesses occur, how they are manifested, and how and why they are cured are a part of many groups, including the medical establishment. Generally, among rural Southerners, health is perceived in terms of maintaining a balance between the good and evil forces in the world. Individuals are always being pulled by these forces and must maintain harmony through their behavior by using available resources in their environment. Medical doctors are just one resource in maintaining this balance. Thus, when a new health program is implemented in rural areas, it is viewed as just one answer to health problems and is usually incorporated into the health behavior of the population. It is not believed to be the only answer to their health problems. Development of health care in the rural South thus involves a translation process between two subcultures—that of the people and that of the health providers (Hill 1980). In a later chapter, I argue that policies and planning for health care delivery systems in the United States should extend beyond the medical system and should be based on a sociocultural model of health: in this case, a model that is culturally appropriate and meaningful to rural Southerners instead of a model which merely maintains or increases the power of those who are dominant in our present political economy.

Until recently, the economic development of the South was secondary to that of the North. Indeed, the North can be seen as the "significant other" to the South (Tindall 1974). Against this background, a distinctive culture has developed and maintained itself which, Tindall feels, is not disappearing. Likewise, I feel that the South has a self-conscious and identifiable culture, and "persists as a coherent collection of assumptions, values, traditions and commitments" (Hill 1977). Many of the symbols that provide meaning for a Southerner are shared; however, social factors (economics and politics) diffuse the uniformity which accounts for overlapping beliefs among different subgroups, producing a heterogeneity based on the differential meanings that occur due to access to different information and to the social structure in general.

Conflicts often arise when economic and political issues (mostly externally controlled), clash with the cultural system of a population. In these situations, ideology and structure are often both integrated, creating continuity, and in conflict, creating change. Ambiguity usually occurs, allowing for different interpretations of goals and events. Generally, the most powerful interpretation prevails, making sense of one group's social situation, but often at the expense of another group. A synthesis of interpretations can occur, however, because some symbols and ideas are shared on various levels within the social structure. Within the Southern context, synthesis often takes the form of paternalism and gives the appearance of continuity for a time. Indeed, Geertz has stated that "ideology bridges the emotional gap between things as they are and as one would have them be . . . The South would not be the South without the existence of popular symbols charged with emotion of a pervasive social predicament" (1975:14). Most of these symbols are those belonging to the "folk tradition," i.e., those of rural peoples who were yeomen farmers, not those of the plantation society whose members were more world-centered.

People cannot escape their history. The threads of a rural Southern past are linked to present experience. The processes that cause conflict arise within the system itself and are creating new patterns. A population is not locked into repetitive traditional patterns. Culture is a creative force; it constitutes as well as being constitutive and provides a means for a population to experience new kinds of consciousness, including health consciousness.

Linking Macro-Micro Levels of Health Policy

A heuristic approach to understanding continuity and change in a complex health system is to separate out the various systems of biology, human activity and ideology into discrete units and analyze the impact one system has on other systems within an environment. This approach assumes that all subsystems are interrelated and that the interaction of one component with another cannot be studied without understanding how all the analytical units fit together. It is an approach that helps us make sense of "organized complexity" (Bertalanffy 1968). A systems approach is an organizational tool that often classifies (albeit frequently simplifies) things among a complex of systems. I prefer to modify a strict systems approach to extend it beyond the ecological model and to include, on an equal basis, the cultural aspects of groups. This means that groups and communities must be analyzed as part of a system, although not necessarily as part of the dominant structure. It is here that anthropologists make a major contribution to the systems approach. They link the microlevel of community to the macrolevel of national/international structure and policies.

Furthermore, systems do not necessarily strain toward equilibrium. Institutions and symbols are sources of order in a social system, but are also the source of conflict as changes occur in people's social and cultural worlds. Therefore, a systems approach does not completely manifest itself toward homeostatis but must incorporate a conflict model of society. This can help us understand and explain how social, cultural, psychological and biological factors converge to on the one hand maintain a continuity, and on the other hand create and explain discontinuities in the human experience.

Several comments need to be made about the approach of this study to exploring the interactions among a rural health system, people and policy. First, no system exists in a vacuum. Although each will be isolated in the various chapters, and some interpreted as more powerful factors than others, it is clear that one system cannot be usefully interpreted without analyzing its links to other systems. As simple as this assumption may sound, the ideas behind a system have both theoretical and empirical significance. Activities and ideas flow from one system to another (in the form of inputs/outputs), influencing and shaping the conditions to which people in the system and the systems themselves must adapt. Consequently, health care systems and people respond to the flow of both new and old activities and ideas (Figure 1). These responses are differential along class lines in Coberly, the community to be considered here, creating a heterogeneity of opportunity among social groups.

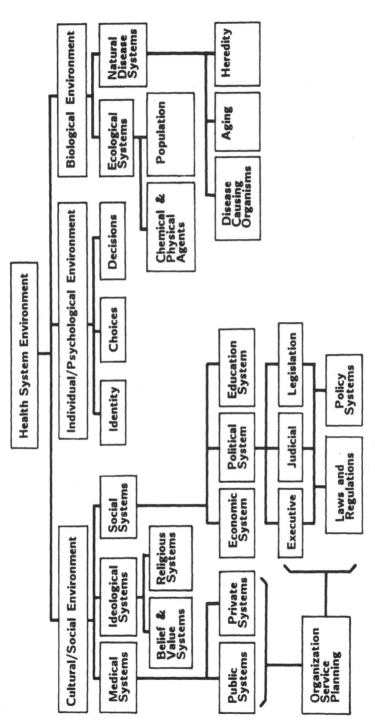

Figure 1. Health System Environment

In this process, each system both accumulates and discards resources in responding to the inputs (potential changes) from other systems. These dynamics are the bases upon which systems persist and change through time. For example, a health system continues to function in Coberly although the content and size of its repertoire changes. Indeed, the boundaries of "health" itself, from a institutional perspective, can be expanded or contracted as health policy changes. A confounding factor, however, in such a straight-forward analysis, and one that the anthropological approach can clear up, relates to the people's view of their health system: the local level analysis (Rodin, et al. 1978). The people of Coberly and the policy-makers have some different views of what constitutes a health system; the meaning of the term "health system" and all its ramifications both converge and diverge in the minds of groups of people on all levels.

Clearly one of the shortcomings of a traditional systems approach is the assumption that all the components of a system, or the units of subsystems, are necessarily working toward a re-establishment of a state of equilibrium. In fact, the people that make up the subsystems do not necessarily perceive the goals of a system in similar fashion. Easton criticizes a traditional systems approach by stating, "It is as though the pathways taken to manage the displacements were an incidental rather than a central theoretical consid-eration" (1965:20). He continues:

> A system may well seek goals other than those of reaching one or another point of equilibrium. Even though this state were to be used only as a theoretical norm that is never achieved, it would offer a less useful theoretical approximation of reality than one that takes into account other possibilties. . . . Furthermore, with respect to these variable goals, it is a primary characteristic that all systems are able to adopt a wide range of actions of a positive, constructive, and innovative sort of warding off or absorbing any forces of displacement. A system need not just react to disturbance by oscillating in the neighborhood of a prior point of equilibrium or by shifting to a new one. It may cope with the disturbances by seeking to change the environment so that exchanges between the environment and itself are no longer stressful; it may seek to insulate itself against any further influences from the environment; or the members of the system may even transform their own relationships fundamentally and modify their own goals and practices so as to improve their chances of handling the inputs from the environment. In these and other ways a system has the capacity for creative and constructive regulation of disturbances. . . . It is clear that the adoption of equilibrium analysis, however latent it may be, obscures the presence of system goals that cannot be described as a state of equilibrium. It also virtually conceals the existence of varying pathways for attaining these alternative ends (1965:20-21).

A key concept for energizing a static traditional systems approach is that of linkage. How and why do the subsystems and systems create links, break links or maintain links in bringing about continuity and change? It is the various linkages of structures, decisions, functions and people that serve to integrate and order the system on both a vertical and a horizontal axis. They provide the vehicle through which inputs and outputs are transmitted via behavior, information, policies and symbols.

These linkages extend from the local community to the national and international level and permeate the boundaries of all the subsystems. These parts of the social system interact in a multidimensional hierarchy; formal and informal, vertical and horizonal, and symmetrical and asymmetrical. The parts are integrated at different levels and feed back into one another on both a micro- and a macro- level. By investigating the different forms of linkages between these levels and analyzing their feedback loops on a particular issue and/or goal, we will be able to delineate more clearly the change process of opposition and synthesis through time (Figure 2).

New forms of articulation between the hierarchical levels are necessary because linkages channel the flow of people and information (Figure 3); thus analyzing the different forms they take, both structurally and ideologically, provides a key for predicting the content of future changes in the system as linkages expand or contract. The formal (organizational) and informal (personal influences) linkages integrate the system in both symmetrical and asymmetrical relationships, implying a reciprocity of benefit among the people, groups, information and policies. These linkages can be activated at different points in the system, from the top down or bottom up. These points become sources for creating opposition (conflict) in the entire cultural and structural system and, through time, function to restructure the formal and informal hierarchical organization. These reorderings occur ideologically as well as structurally as long as some goals and structure are shared and cultural models converge on some axis. In establishing both continuity and change (as the studies and culture change), the system will often appear ambiguous, providing the basis for a multitude of interpretations and, consequently, differentiation of social groups in the system. This differentiation process is inextricably bound to the hegemony of the economic and political system in the U.S.

Policy is viewed as similar to a kinship system, a religious system, or a health system; it is both a social and a cultural system. The meaning that shapes reality within the health policy area provides guidelines for instituting behavioral and structural changes. Indeed, culture mediates between the points of intersection of the health policy system. It thereby shapes the policy reality within the multilayered structure of the health policy system, which for analytical purposes is somewhat artifical and in reality cannot be fully understood without connecting it to the systems of the whole. Gil (1970) and De Miquel (1975) argue for a holistic approach to policy and

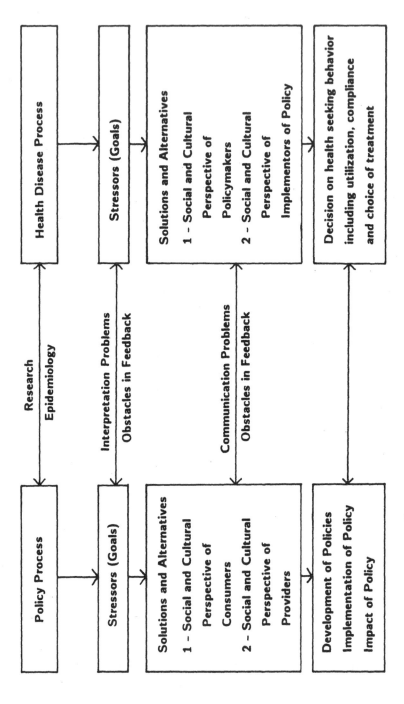

Figure 2. Variables Involved on Macro and Micro Levels

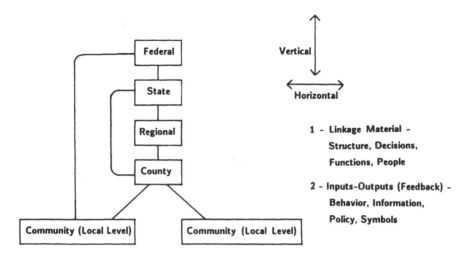

Figure 3. Linkage Chains

feel that we need to understand the "whole" impact that policy decisions have on one another by analyzing all the dynamic processes of society.

Studies in the past decade have pointed out a variety of factors that influence the health system. For example, the Health Field Concept put forth by La Londe (1974) pointed out that four major variables are responsible for the health status of populations: biology, environment, lifestyle and health services. His model is in accordance with the writings of McKeown (1975), who demonstrated that the factors responsible for the modern improvement in health status are mainly behavioral and environmental. He feels that the effects of immunization and therapy have been recent and relatively small and that today, health is determined mainly by lifestyle. According to the Surgeon Generals' Report on Health Promotion and Disease Prevention, "Many of today's most pressing 'health problems' are related to excesses—of smoking, drinking, faulty nutrition, overuse of medication, fast driving, and relentless pressure to achieve" (U.S. Department of Health, Education and Welfare 1979). The report calculates that almost half of U.S. mortality in 1976 was due to unhealthy behavior or lifestyle, 20% to environmental factors, 20% to human biological factors and 10% to inadequacies in health care. These factors, then, are unequal in their impact on health in general and on specific populations in a community.

Likewise, Blum (1976) views health from a general systems approach which posits that systems are able to resist or overcome forces which threaten to disrupt their functioning, either internally or through commanding support from other systems via feedback loops (Figure 4). Systems, however, because they adapt to disturbances are in a constant state of

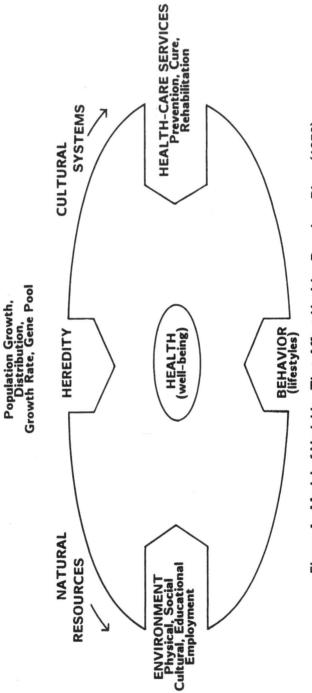

Figure 4. Model of Variables That Affect Health. Based on Blum (1976).
Note: These variables are called "Major Risk Categories.

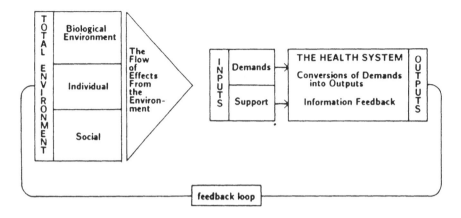

Figure 5. A Response Model of a Health System

change. These disturbances (including all of the other systems) originate in the environment and provide a stimulus that may strain the system, although it does not necessarily do so. In the health system, physical and mental illnesses are forces that stress or disrupt either the entire system or one of several levels and demand a response. The causes of illnesses and disease arise then from disturbance in the system/subsystems and provide inputs and outputs between the environment, the health system, and individuals in a population. It is when stress is believed to occur that interventions are planned and implemented. New and/or old linkages are activated in an attempt to counteract the negative inputs with positive inputs that will allow the system to adapt. These structures, decisions, people and functions vary according to how serious or threatening the stress or disruption is perceived to be, the nature of the resources necessary to respond to the stress, and the population that is experiencing stress (Figure 5).

In this book, these processes are analyzed on the local level, in the community of Coberly. Since policies are guidelines for social development, we first need to understand the forces in Coberly that maintain and change the health systems of the community. Thus, its social order is described as well as the mechanisms (linkages) of social change. An analysis such as this must consider both the social and ideological aspects of the community as they relate to health and the social and ideological aspects of the health policy on all levels. Health policy is, then, only one component of the health system and forms a subsystem itself that differentially impacts communities and groups in a community. The factors that explain such differentiation are explored in this book with a detailed analysis of Coberly; a complicating aspect of this analysis is the community's heterogeneity. On the local level of community, the cultural and structural components of the policy systems link differently with the different components of the community systems. Their feedback into the other systems (the level notwithstanding) becomes apparent when we examine the major variables that impinge upon the health status of a population.

In Coberly, we shall examine both the community health system and the health policy system, and their subsystems, in the context of culture and structure. This type of study serves as an ethnographic example of how the systems approach can integrate levels of analysis, both theoretically and empirically. Furthermore, this approach provides a mechanism through which the microlevel of community health culture and structure can be analytically combined with the macrolevel of the structure and culture of policy. The policy level is viewed as the external system of medicine that sets conditions for health action (practice) in the community of Coberly but does not determine it. I hope to demonstrate how people participate in creating their own transformations and in doing so, are not just reactors to the medical system. Ortner in her assessment of anthropological theory in the 1980's states that "The newer practice theorists [however] share a view that 'the system' does in fact have a very powerful, even 'determining' effect upon human action and the shape of events" although "questions concerning these relationships may go in either direction—the impact of the system on practice, and the impact of practice on the system" (1984:146-148).

Development of Health Care in the Rural South

Public health services in the rural South have been, until recently, the major health services available to most rural peoples, unless there happened to be a private white doctor in the area. The first full-time county health department in the South was established in Jefferson County, Kentucky in 1908 and the second in Guilford, North Carolina in 1911. Funds for these facilities became available through passage of one of the first federal laws that placed special emphasis on studying rural areas, the Rural Sanitation Act of 1916—a part of the Field Investigations of Public Health. Programs were carried out in rural areas in Maryland and Indiana during the summers of 1914 and 1916 in which public health workers gave advice about the safe disposal of human wastes, the protection of water supplies, and screening against insects. Associated programs dramatically lowered the rate for typhoid fever (Williams 1951). Studies at this time found that: (1) less than two percent of the homes consistently practiced the principle of sanitation; (2) fewer than three percent were served adequately by local health services; (3) sustained efficient and full-time local health services were essential to the establishment of good sanitary conditions; and (4) efficient personnel could not be expected, without active participation in the work of central agencies, to prevent the adverse influence of local politics (Schmeckebrer 1923).

Furthermore, during this time, a study conducted to delineate the kind of county health unit needed in rural areas concluded that sufficient funds and qualified personnel, as well as office space, furniture, records, clerical staff and transportation for official purposes were needed to maintain an effective unit (Williams 1951). In 1919, one of the first studies in industrial preventive medicine in the South, (requested by the Central of Georgia Railroad), found that a substantial loss of time from work by employees was due to malaria. Consequently, the railroad undertook drainage and screening work for the protection of its employees. Other companies followed these preventive practices.

In the following decades, we find that public health services in rural areas continued to focus their efforts on malaria control and community sanitation. These efforts included the construction of sanitary privies and the sealing of abandoned mines. For example, in 1934, the Federal Emergency Relief Administration allocated one million dollars to the Public Health Service for rural health work. In 1935, the Public Health Service assigned medical personnel to furnish health guidance for programs that were being developed by the Farm Security Administration. They began to attack what they deemed the major problem facing rural families—the lack of adequate medical care. Subsequently, many programs of rural rehabilitation developed active medical care, which they felt would improve the financial condition and economic rehabilitation of rural areas (Williams 1951).

In the 1930s, 1940s, and 1950s, three major health programs that affected health care in the South were implemented. The Center for Disease Control was created mainly to control infectious disease, especially malaria in the South. It worked with state public health programs to improve the health of Southerners. Beginning in the 1920s, and through the 1940s, most Southern states began midwifery programs. Lay midwives were trained by local and state health departments to make home deliveries. These programs targeted poor people who could not afford medical care.

Another program, Hill-Burton, was established in 1947 and provided matching federal funds for hospital construction and modernization. Two decades later, short-stay, nonfederal beds had increased by 41 percent. Most of the Hill-Burton funds, however, were concentrated in urban areas, and thus began the era of hospital-based specialized medical care. At the same time, the number of family practice physicians decreased, leaving small towns with physician shortages (Decker 1977). Hill-Burton also contributed to the excess of physical facilities in rural areas (Kane 1977).

In the 1960s, efforts to provide adequate hospitalization were continued, while programs such as Medicare and Medicaid were established for the purpose of defraying the medical expenses of the poor, large percentages of whom live in rural areas in the South. In addition, the Office of Economic Opportunity, part of the War on Poverty, initiated a variety of programs to provide health care for the poor.

In the 1970s, the Rural Health Initiative Projects Bill was passed and began to be administered by the Public Health Service. Its purpose was to develop and systematize the delivery of health care in rural areas. The several programs included under this act are: (1) National Health Service Corps, (2) Community Health Centers, (3) Migrant Health Programs, (4) Health Underserved Rural Areas Programs and (5) Appalachian Health Programs. The goal of these programs was to provide primary health care for rural areas. This has resulted in clinics being constructed in small towns. Consequently, in the late 1970s, rural areas experienced the effects of governmental policies' attempting to change the health status of rural peoples.

These efforts notwithstanding, we find that rural people continue to have limited access to mainstream medical resources, and that their health status is among the worst in the nation. Recent statistics show that the poor and undereducated still utilize health services less than other groups. This under-utilization is due to inability to afford services, lack of available information about mainstream medicine, and different ideas about illness and health (Bergner and Yerby 1976).

The poor health status of rural Southerners is not the result of either economic factors or cultural factors alone, or merely a combination of them. The answer is more complicated. It involves the unique society/state relationship created by historical, political, economic and cultural factors. The culture of one social group, (i.e., policy-makers), does not necessarily provide a readymade set of solutions to the problems of another social group (rural Southerners). The efforts of policy-makers to provide adequate medical care to rural areas are based on their model of health and devoting attention to individuals rather than on the economic and political origins of illness.

From this wider perspective, it seems to me that a broad health care delivery system is the first step toward creating new meanings for rural Southerners. Access is a process in which decisions are made by both policy-makers and the people themselves. And we find that when a health care program cannot meet the goals, both of the granting agencies, and of the existing economic, social and political structures in the community, it is more than likely doomed to fail. This process is convincingly illustrated by Couto (1975) in his study of the Floyd County Comprehensive Health Service Program in eastern Kentucky. The failure of that program was not due to "culture" but to the conflicts that arose over who controlled the clinics and who interpreted the meaning of health.

Rural Health Care

As we moved into the 1980's, rural areas accounted for 32 percent of the nation's population, almost 50 percent of the nation's poor, and 39 percent of the nation's elderly and children. Yet rural people receive less than 25 percent of all Medicaid funds, and the rural elderly obtain only 29 percent of funds for hospital and post-hospital care. In addition, only 23 percent of federal and state expenditures on maternal and child health programs go to rural areas, while 75 percent of all neighborhood health centers are in urban areas. Lastly, we find that the programs designated to improve rural health have been funded at very low levels (Davis and Marshall 1979).

Money from governmental projects related to rural health or to actual health problems of rural people, we find, seems to be lacking and, in some cases, almost nonexistent. Low incomes, poor diets, inadequate housing, impure water supplies, poor transportation and communication systems, and limited medical resources are factors which, when combined, are important in explaining the epidemiology of rural areas. It should be pointed out that analysts have some difficulty in establishing either the absolute or the relative health status of people in rural areas. In addition to data problems, many find it difficult to decide which indicators are best for describing overall health status (Gilford et al., 1981).

These problems notwithstanding, we find that, based on single indices or a composite index, the health status of rural people is worse than that of any other population (Ahearn 1979). Similar findings are reported by Copp (1976), who identified several predominantly rural groups that have disproportionately severe health needs. They include Southern rural Blacks, Chicanos, Appalachian and Ozark Whites, the aged migrant workers, illegal aliens and residents of environmentally polluted areas. They all share the characteristics of being poor, powerless and discriminated against because of race, culture or lifestyle.

Specifically, rural areas have four times the national rate for accidents. The infant mortality rate among the rural poor is 20 percent higher than among the urban poor and 50 percent higher than the national rate. Among poor rural Blacks, the infant mortality rate is double the national average. Chronic conditions are more prevalent among rural residents of all ages: pleurisy, arthritis, rheumatism, emphysema, hypertensive heart disease and cerebrovascular disease (Table 1). Of all the new cases of tuberculosis, 54 percent are in rural areas. And the life expectancy of migrant farmworkers is 49 years, 23 years less than the national average (Davis and Marshall 1979).

A major factor in understanding rural health is the general problem of access to health care, which according to health planners reflects the

TABLE 1

Incidence of Selected Chronic Conditions (rates per 1,000 population, by place of residence, U.S., selected years between 1968 and 1972)

	U.S.	SMSA	Non-SMSA	Ratio, Non-SMSA to SMSA
Conditions relatively more prevalent in nonmetropolitan areas				
Chronic digestive conditions				
Ulcer of stomach & duodenum	17.2	15.9	19.4	1.22
Upper GI disorders	13.1	11.7	15.6	1.33
Gallbladder	10.3	9.0	12.6	1.40
Constipation	23.8	20.9	28.9	1.21
Chronic respiratory conditions				
Emphysema	6.6	5.4	8.7	1.61
Sinusitis	103.0	96.3	115.3	1.20
Pleurisy	3.4	2.9	4.5	1.55
Chronic circulatory conditions				
Hypertensive heart disease	10.5	9.6	12.1	1.26
Cerebrovascular disease	7.5	6.8	8.8	1.29
Chronic skin and musculoskeletal conditions				
Disease of nails	22.9	20.2	29.3	1.40
Arthritis	92.9	86.0	106.2	1.23
Rheumatism	6.1	5.2	7.8	1.50
Displaced disc	8.6	8.0	9.6	1.20
Conditions relatively more prevalent in metropolitan areas				
Chronic respiratory conditions				
Deflected nasal septum	4.0	5.2	1.8	.35
Laryngitis	5.7	6.3	4.8	.76
Chronic circulatory conditions				
Congenital abnormalities	4.4	4.9	3.6	.73
Chronic skin and musculoskeletal conditions				
Psoriasis	6.5	7.1	5.3	.75
Gout	4.8	5.2	4.1	.79

Source: U.S. Department of Health, Education, and Welfare, National Center for Health Statistics. Prevalence of Selected Chronic Digestive Conditions, U.S., July–December 1968, Series 10, No. 83; Prevalence of Chronic Skin and Musculoskeletal Conditions, U.S. 1969, Series 10, No. 92; Prevalence of Selected Chronic Respiratory Conditions, U.S. 1970, Series 10, No. 84; Prevalence of Chronic Circulatory Conditions, U.S. 1972, Series 10, No. 94

distribution of health resources. There is clearly a discrepancy between rural and urban population-to-health personnel ratios. Indeed, we find that approximately 49 million people reside in "medically underserved areas" of which 29 million or about 60 percent, are rural dwellers. Similarly, over 950 counties have been identified as having critical health personnel shortages, with 84 percent of these being rural counties. While the rural population makes up 32 percent of the nation's population, it is served by only 12 percent of the nation's physicians and 18 percent of its nurses (Rural America 1977). Thus, there is a strong negative relationship between the total number of physicians and the degree of rurality of their location for practice, a pattern that also holds true for other medical personnel (Cordes 1976; Ahearn 1979). On the other hand, the distribution of mid-level health personnel is generally more even. Almost half (46.1 percent) of Physician's Assistants work in areas with a population of less than 50,000 (Perry and Fisher 1980).

The general distribution of health facilities reflects a more positive picture for rural areas. In 1976, there were 495 U.S. counties without a community hospital, the majority of which were in rural areas. There were, however, more community hospitals per capita in rural areas than in urban areas. Rural people use hospitals more often than urban people and are injured less (Ahearn 1979). They use them for a wider range of problems than urban dwellers. Nursing homes are less available, however, to the rural elderly than to the urban elderly, although the rural elderly almost double the urban elderly in number. In 1975, there were 479 nursing home beds per 100,000 people in urban areas as compared to 407 in rural areas (Ahearn 1979).

Although the rural middle class and blue-collar workers tend to utilize the medical system more often and generally comply with its directives more readily than the poor, the general rural environment, its overall economic status and geographic barriers affect their health status also. Together, all social strata and ethnic groups (Black and White) participate in a medical system in which there is limited availability of health professionals and poor communication and transportation services. Primary preventive services, particularly for children and women, are frequently neglected. Services providing prenatal care, cancer screening, and contraceptive information are underutilized.

Most rural people also share the same water and sewer system (although the extension of these services to Blacks and outside the small town is a relatively recent development), or rely on wells and/or outdoor bathrooms. Consequently, dental problems due to the lack of fluoridated water sources are widespread, as are bacterial and parasitic diseases. The lack of solid waste disposal also creates a higher risk for contaminated water supplies and infections, and some rural areas experience pollution from fertilizer, pesticides and mining. Lastly, most rural areas have limited economic opportunities, cultural and recreational resources and, as a consequence, have a higher rate of mental health problems such as alcoholism and depression (Davis and Marshall 1979). These health status factors of rural people provided an impetus for the federal government to pass legislation aimed at improving the health status of a large sector of the nation's population.

The concept of "medically underserved populations" began with the Health Maintenance Organization Act of 1973, which required that funding priorities be given to Health Maintenance Organizations (HMO's) serving "medically underserved populations." Both urban and rural areas can be designated as underserved, although more rural areas by far have qualified for priority funding. In the American South, the situation is critical, and the North Georgia town of Coberly—the subject of this study—reflects the general problems related to rural health. Indeed, as we shall see, Coberly qualified as a medically underserved area, and as a consequence, has a new primary health care clinic.

Race, Health, and Poverty in the South

In most rural areas of the South, we can best understand health care in terms of race and poverty. Statistical data from the past twenty years demonstrate that the poor, undereducated, and Blacks visit doctors less frequently than other groups and thus underutilize the mainstream medical system. Karpatkin has stated that:

> our health-care system provides inadequate insurance protection to the poor and the financing of health services is drastic and often emotional . . . the present system results in a lower quality of health care for the poor than for the well-to-do, is cost-inefficient, and leaves both enlightened physicians and many consumers of its services dissatisfied (1976:44).

The reasons for this underutilization, and for lack of compliance with the advice of health care providers, vary according to the comprehensive state program and the degree of isolation of communities. They generally, however, include the inability to afford services, problems with transportation, different definitions of illness, and limited access to information about the mainstream medical system. In addition, the poor are less likely to use preventive measures, and are more likely to select paraprofessionals or lay practitioners, and generally delay seeking medical help (Bergner and Yerby 1976).

In 1970, 41.2 percent of Southerners were rural dwellers, as compared to 26.5 percent nationwide. Excluding Florida, more than 47 percent of the South was rural, with the states of Mississippi, North Carolina, and

TABLE 2
Poverty Rates for Families by Race and Residence in the South (1970)
(in percentages)

	Total	White	Black
Urbanized Areas			
Central Cities	15	9	32
Urban Fringe	8	6	29
Other Urban			
10,000 – 49,999	16	11	41
2,500 – 9,999	18	13	45
Rural	23	17	52

Source: Gretchen Maclachlan, *The Other Twenty Percent: A Statistical Analysis of Poverty in the South* (Southern Regional Council, Inc., Atlanta, GA, 1974), p. 7.

South Carolina having over 50 percent rural population. The rural poor account for a large part of the 1976 statistics on household income in the South. Twenty-five percent of the nation's population lives in the South and accounts for 38 percent of the nation's poor. In 1977, 20.7 percent of household annual incomes in the South were under $1500, with the average income for all households being $11,591. The median annual income for the region was $12,562, only 84 percent of the nation's median income level, while the average individual income level was 33 percent of the national average at $3756. (It is thought by many health planners that household income is a more meaningful economic indicator than individual income, since the proportion of nuclear family households is decreasing while the number of households composed of unrelated individuals is increasing [Rogers 1979]). Furthermore, the percentage of poor families headed by females is far greater than those headed by males in the the South. Although a majority of Southern poor work, they do not earn enough to raise their income above the poverty level (Maclachlan 1974). Rogers feels that "the level of family income in a population group is the most influential characteristic which determines whether that population will have health services which are appropriate and accessible" (Rogers 1979:4).

Not surprisingly, we find that the poverty rate for the South in 1970 was more than 40 percent higher than the national rate—23 percent of the 25 million people in the South lived in poverty (Table 2). In 1975, 51.6 percent of black children, ages 5–17, lived in homes below the poverty level. Statistics for the following year, 1976, indicate that 16.6 percent of people (black and white) in the South lived in poverty, while 35.8 percent of Blacks in the region were below the poverty level, as compared to 31.1 percent in the nation. When income is computed for families, we find that 13.2 percent of Blacks and Whites in the South were below the poverty level in the 1970's while 31.8 percent of black families lived below the poverty level (Rogers 1979). In absolute terms, more poor families are headed by white males, but the incidence of poverty is highest among black female-headed families. Overall, 2 out of 3 Southern families are poor. Over 50 percent of Blacks in rural areas are poor and about 17 percent of Whites are poor in the South (Tables 3, 4). The Southern Regional Council reports that these figures have not changed substantially in the past ten years (Southern Regional Council 1986).

The epidemiological patterns among rural black and white Southerners are indicators of the health status of the population and when compared to national patterns reflect rather serious problems. Nationwide, the annual death rate among Blacks is nearly 50 percent higher than among Whites. The average life expectancy for Blacks in the U.S. is 65.3 years, while for Whites it is 71.7 years. Life expectancy also varies sharply by sex and age within these groups (Table 5), in accordance with mortality rates on a nationwide basis (Table 6). In short, according to available statistics, Blacks have a shorter life expectancy by seven to eight years than Whites, with a particularly high mortality rate between the ages of 55 and 69. Furthermore, black men have significantly higher death rates from heart attack (316.7 per 100,000 compared to 268.8 for white men), stroke (72.7 per 100,000 compared to 38.9 for white men), lung cancer (84.1 per 100,000 compared to 57.8 for white men), and cancer of the digestive tract (Human Services Annual Report 1984).

In the South, both infant and general mortality rates are substantially higher than in other regions of the country. Davis and Marshall report that:

> In 1971, infant mortality rates in the non-metropolitan, 13-state South were 23.3 deaths per 1000 live births compared with 19.0 per 1000 nationally, or 23% higher than the national average infant mortality rate. General mortality rates were also higher in the non-metropolitan South, averaging 11.3 deaths per 1000 population compared with 8.5 per 1000 in the metropolitan South and 9.3 per 1000 nationally. Thus, the general death rates were 22 percent higher in the non-metropolitan South than the metropolitan South (1979:66).

With regard to ethnic differences, they note that infant mortality rates among rural Southern Blacks are 65 percent higher than among rural Southern Whites, and infant mortality rates for both groups are higher in rural counties. These rates are also higher in counties with higher incidences of poverty, as are general mortality rates. Furthermore, the morbidity and disability rates are higher in the rural South, with more bed disability among the elderly. Although children have a lower incidence of respiratory and infectious diseases, adults have a higher rate of acute conditions, especially injuries. In fact, in 1976, the rate of bed disability was 16 percent

TABLE 3
Families by Race and Residence: Poverty Rates (1970) (in percentages)

	Urban					
	Central Cities	Urban Fringe	10,000–49,999	2,500–9,999	Rural	Total
Alabama						
White	7.6	7.1	10.8	13.2	19.4	13.6
Black	38.7	36.9	43.0	48.3	58.2	46.7
Arkansas						
White	8.8	9.0	11.7	15.9	23.4	17.7
Black	40.4	42.0	50.5	53.4	60.2	52.7
Florida						
White	9.2	6.8	8.5	11.2	13.7	9.5
Black	33.5	27.5	40.3	42.1	47.4	36.3
Georgia						
White	8.9	4.4	9.6	10.9	14.4	10.5
Black	31.0	24.8	41.4	45.0	51.5	39.7
Louisiana						
White	8.5	6.4	12.7	13.4	18.9	12.6
Black	40.2	35.1	48.8	51.9	59.0	47.4
Mississippi						
White	8.7	7.2	10.3	12.6	20.8	15.9
Black	40.4	44.9	50.7	54.8	66.7	59.2
North Carolina						
White	6.4	7.5	8.4	10.1	13.6	11.1
Black	30.1	22.2	35.5	40.0	44.8	38.7
South Carolina						
White	8.3	8.6	8.3	8.9	12.3	10.5
Black	40.2	31.3	36.6	40.5	50.0	44.7
Tennessee						
White	7.6	4.9	12.2	15.1	21.7	15.3
Black	34.0	35.9	37.6	40.6	51.1	38.0
Texas						
White	10.8	5.2	13.5	17.0	18.4	12.4
Black	27.2	26.6	35.7	44.6	50.2	32.7
Virginia						
White	7.4	4.1	7.7	8.1	14.3	9.0
Black	27.0	20.6	23.4	31.1	36.4	29.9
11-State South						
White	9.2	5.8	10.7	13.0	17.0	12.0
Black	32.4	29.3	41.3	45.3	52.1	41.0

Source: Gretchen Maclachlan, The Other Twenty Percent: A Statistical Analysis of Poverty in the South (Southern Regional Council, Inc., Atlanta, GA, 1974), p. 7.

TABLE 4

POVERTY INCIDENCE IN THE SOUTH FOR FAMILIES BY RACE,
SEX, AND RESIDENCE OF FAMILY HEAD (1970)

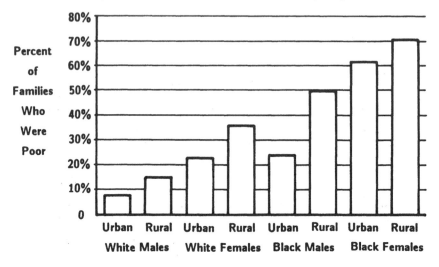

Source: Maclachlan, Gretchen, The Other Twenty Percent: A
        Statistical Analysis of Poverty in the South, Southern
        Regional Council, Inc., Atlanta, GA, 1974, p. 7.

TABLE 5
Differences in Life Expectancy by Race, Age, and Sex (1981)

Age	White		Black	
	Male	Female	Male	Female
0	71.1	78.5	64.4	73.0
10	62.2	69.4	56.2	64.7
20	52.7	59.7	46.6	54.9
30	43.5	50.0	37.9	45.4
40	34.2	40.4	29.5	36.3
50	25.4	31.2	22.0	27.8
60	17.7	22.7	15.8	20.3
70	11.5	15.1	10.8	13.9
80	6.9	8.9	6.5	8.4

Source: USDHHS/PHS, National Center for Health Statistics 1986, Vital Statistics
of the United States, 1981. Vol. 2—Mortality. Part A. Washington, D.C.: U.S.
Government Printing Office.

higher in the South than the national rate; the percentage of people limited
in activity due to chronic conditions was 12 percent higher, and the
percentage with disabilities that render a person unable to carry out major
activities 34 percent higher (Rogers 1979). Nutritional levels are also lower,
and the incidence of most chronic conditions is greater (hypertensive heart

TABLE 6
Differences in Mortality Rates by Race and Age (per thousand) 1972

Age	Black	White	Differences
0–15	0.9	0.6	0.3
15–34	2.9	1.3	1.6
35–54	9.8	4.5	5.3
55–69	24.9	15.5	9.8
70–79	58.6	53.8	4.8
80+	99.0	134.9	–35.8
All Ages	9.3	9.4	–0.1

Source: National Center for Health Statistics, U.S. Department of Health, Education, and Welfare, Vol. 20, 1972.

TABLE 7
Total Numbers of Black Physicians by State: Total and in Rural Counties

State	Total Number Physicians	Total Number Black Physicians	Number Black Physicians in Rural Counties
Alabama	3,143	70	23
Arkansas	1,845	19	2
Florida	11,216	99	2
Georgia	5,141	117	17
Louisiana	4,478	66	2
Mississippi	1,838	56	12
North Carolina	5,694	141	34
South Carolina	2,468	53	31
Tennessee	4,833	204	10
Texas	13,462	182	6
Virginia	5,850	152	12

Source: *Health Care in the South: A Statistical Profile*, Southern Regional Council, 1975.

disease, cerebrovascular heart disease, ulcers, emphysema, arthritis and rheumatism).

Additional statistics indicate further problems in rural areas. For example, there are fewer patient care physicians per capita than in other areas, fewer physician services and more hospital stays. According to Davis and Marshall (1979) " . . . since residents of the non-metropolitan South have a higher incidence of health problems, they would appear to be under-utilizers of ambulatory health services relative to their urban counterparts with similar health status" (1979:68). Lastly, dental visits in the rural South are 65 percent lower than in the urban South. Generally, then, we find that health care services in the rural areas of the South are inadequate (Wheeler 1976).

Conditions are worse among rural Blacks, where the lack of black physicians is acute (Table 7). According to Davis and Marshall (1979), this shortage may be of increased significance in Southern rural areas where Blacks (denied the opportunity to utilize black physicians) still see white physicians in white clinics, are still segregated in waiting rooms and restricted to certain hours of access in some areas and even lack knowledge about the medical process. As a result, in general, rural Blacks tend to underutilize existing medical facilities as compared with rural Whites (Salber, et al. 1976). Thus, although rural Blacks are exposed to most of the same environmental conditions as rural Whites, they consult physicians less frequently. This utilization pattern, combined with the living conditions of poverty, results in a difference in epidemiological patterns for rural Blacks and rural Whites.

The difference in disease patterns cannot be completely explained by differential utilization of medical facilities however, and a more detailed examination of disease patterns is necessary to clarify and explain the differences between the two ethnic groups. We find that two major kinds of diseases among rural Southern Blacks are cardiovascular diseases (hypertensive heart disease, cerebrovascular disease, and arteriosclerosis) and cancer (Table 8). A third category of genetically-linked diseases, like sickle-cell anemia, includes entities unique to the Black population and thus of potential interest. These three groups of illnesses are considered as having a particular impact on the rural black community, and thus present special problems for health care delivery.

Diseases of the heart are the leading cause of death among both Blacks and Whites in the U.S. (Table 9). In 1940, there were fewer deaths from heart disease in the rural South than in the urban South, with 281.9 deaths per 100,000 in rural areas as compared with 444.1 deaths per 100,000 in urban areas (Pennell and Lehman 1951). In urban areas, heart mortality was higher in the North than in the South for each race, except for "the high death rate among negroes and white males in the smaller cities and towns of the South" (1951:61). In a comparison of North-South differences in specific forms of heart disease, Pennell and Lehman found that the Northern mortality rates from diseases of the myocardium were double the Southern rates, and from coronary arteriosclerosis, mortality rates were 59 percent greater in Northern males and 31 percent greater in Northern females.

A study in 1968 found that hypertensive and cerebrovascular heart disease are more prevalent in rural areas across age groups. Hypertensive heart disease is particularly severe among Blacks, and a conservative estimate is that it affects 20 percent of the population (Saunders and Williams 1975:334). Higher Black mortality rates from hypertensive heart disease are found in the East, South, Central and South Atlantic geographic areas, along with greater differences between mortality rates for Blacks and Whites. Indeed, Saunders and Williams state that hypertension among Blacks " . . . develops at an earlier age than among Whites, is frequently more severe and results in a higher mortality at an earlier age, more commonly from stroke than from coronary arterial disease" (1975:334).

TABLE 8
Major Causes of Death Among Blacks in U.S., 1950–1983

Race, sex, and cause of death				Year				
	1950	1960	1970	1979	1980	1981	1982	1983
Black male	Deaths per 100,000 resident population							
All causes	1,373.1	1,246.1	1,318.6	1,073.3	1,112.8	1,067.7	1,045.5	1,024.7
Diseases of heart	415.5	381.2	375.9	314.1	327.3	316.7	—	—
Cerebrovascular diseases	146.2	141.2	124.2	77.9	77.5	72.7	—	—
Malignant neoplasms	126.1	158.5	198.0	221.8	229.9	232.0	—	—
Respiratory system	16.9	36.6	60.8	78.7	82.0	84.1	—	—
Digestive system	59.4	60.4	58.9	60.7	62.1	62.1	—	—
Pneumonia and influenza	63.8	70.2	53.8	24.2	28.0	26.4	—	—
Chronic liver disease and cirrhosis	8.8	14.8	33.1	30.3	30.6	27.3	—	—
Diabetes mellitus	11.5	16.2	21.2	17.0	17.7	16.8	—	—
Accidents and adverse effects	105.7	100.0	119.5	81.3	82.0	74.7	—	—
Motor vehicle accidents	39.8	38.2	50.1	33.7	32.9	30.7	—	—
Suicide	7.0	7.8	9.9	12.5	11.1	11.0	—	—
Homocide and legal intervention	51.1	44.9	82.1	70.1	71.9	69.2	—	—
Black female	Deaths per 100,000 resident population							
All causes	1,106.7	916.9	814.4	605.0	631.1	599.1	570.9	571.5
Diseases of heart	349.5	292.6	251.7	190.9	201.1	191.2	—	—
Cerebrovascular diseases	155.6	139.5	107.9	60.9	61.7	58.1	—	—
Malignant neoplasms	131.9	127.8	123.5	125.1	129.7	127.1	—	—
Respiratory system	4.1	5.5	10.9	17.4	19.5	20.1	—	—
Digestive system	40.2	37.5	34.1	35.0	35.4	34.5	—	—
Breast	19.3	21.3	21.5	22.7	23.3	23.7	—	—
Pneumonia and influenza	50.4	43.9	29.2	10.9	12.7	11.3	—	—
Chronic liver disease and cirrhosis	5.7	8.9	17.8	13.3	14.4	12.7	—	—
Diabetes mellitus	22.7	27.3	30.9	20.8	22.1	21.3	—	—
Accidents and adverse effects	38.5	35.9	35.3	23.9	25.1	21.6	—	—
Motor vehicle accidents	10.3	10.0	13.8	8.7	8.4	7.7	—	—
Suicide	1.7	1.9	2.9	2.9	2.4	2.5	—	—
Homocide and legal intervention	11.7	11.8	15.0	13.9	13.7	12.9	—	—

Source: National Center for Health Statistics, DHHS Publication No. (PHS) 85-1232, 1984.

TABLE 9
Rates of Death from Hypertension by Race, Sex and Age
(per 100,000 population: 1959–61)

Sex and Geographical Area	All Ages	35–44	45–54	55–64	65–74	75–84	85+
White male							
South Atlantic	32.8	6.0	24.5	77.9	200.6	547.9	1,234.2
East South Central	33.2	4.7	20.4	70.7	200.1	615.9	1,409.2
Black male							
South Atlantic	126.0	81.3	195.5	418.3	708.9	931.9	1,540.4
East South Central	106.8	72.5	149.4	333.1	596.2	940.1	1,527.3
White female							
South Atlantic	29.6	3.6	15.1	49.2	180.6	606.6	1,433.6
East South Central	29.4	3.4	14.7	47.9	172.8	629.6	1,400.7
Black female							
South Atlantic	117.4	73.7	174.8	417.8	635.6	875.4	1,472.2
East South Central	106.4	70.9	160.3	328.0	550.7	950.4	1,639.4

Source: I. M. Moriyama et al., Cardiovascular Disease in the U.S. (Cambridge: Harvard University Press, 1971).

Other studies (e.g., McDonough 1964; Howard 1971; Moriyama 1971; Eckenfels 1977; Schoenberger 1975) have documented the striking differences in the rates of hypertension among Blacks and Whites, particularly in the Southern United States. Since this is a "symptomless" disease, medical detection occurs only by means of blood pressure measurement, with the result that large numbers of persons go unscreened and untreated. These people may later develop a number of related complications, including myocardial defects, cerebrovascular disease and renal failure.

The incidence of another disease, cancer, appears to be increasing among rural Blacks. Twenty years ago cancer rates were 20 percent lower for Blacks than for Whites (Lefall 1975). Yet a more recent study by Burbank and Fraumeni shows an increase in the Black-to-White ratio of age-adjusted death rates. They report that non-white predominance began in 1950 for females and in 1956 for males. In females the shift resulted from a decline in death rates among whites, as rates for non-whites remained unchanged; and in males from rates which rose over time in both races but more rapidly in non-whites (1972:649). There is some question as to how much of this increase reflects reporting bias and how much actual increase.

As stated earlier, overall cancer rates are increasing in the South. For example, lung cancer is greatly increasing in both Blacks and Whites, while cancers of the pancreas, prostate, and larynx are also on the rise. Lefall (1975:745) has suggested that the increases in cancer deaths among Blacks may not reflect higher incidences of the disease but errors in reportage in previous years. He also notes that genetic differences in cancer mortality are most sharply reflected in the lack of skin cancer in Blacks due to the presence of melanin, and in higher rates of increase in leukemia and malignant lymphomas among Blacks. Additional research has focused on possible environmental determinants. The most obvious example of such a factor is cigarette smoking's relationship to increases in cancers of the lung, larynx, mouth, esophagus, pancreas and bladder (Burbank and Fraumeni 1972:657). Other environmental carcinogens may also be involved, particularly from exposure levels inherent in certain occupations. Lefall further notes that other types of cancer, like carcinoma of the cervix, may be directly associated with certain socio-economic conditions such as early sexual exposure and frequent childbirth (1975:758). Cancer again is an example of a disease with a complex basis. As Burbank and Fraumeni concluded that "clear-cut differences in cancer risk among widely separate black populations indicate the activity of environmental carcinogens in both continents. On the other hand, genetic factors may be responsible for racial variation in some cancers since rates among U.S. whites are much higher than among blacks in either the U.S. or Africa" (1972:657). Sickle-cell anemia is the one disease of Blacks specifically known to be genetically determined. The relationship of sickle-cell polymorphia to restricted oc-curences of falciparum malaria has been well documented. Research interest in the disease has led directly to greater success in recent years in screening and controlling it. Darity (1977) has reported that one out of every 500 Blacks has the sickle-cell disease, with an additional 2 million carrying the genes. The latest statistics on incidence of chronic illnesses do not break down into SMSA and Non-SMSA. They do, however, report that chronic sinusitis is ranked first among Whites while hypertensive disease is ranked first among Blacks. Arthritis is ranked second among both Blacks and Whites (DHHS 1986).

Black Southerners

About one third of the Black population of the South is rural, with Arkansas, Mississippi and the Carolinas being the only states in which over half the Black population is classified as rural. In 1970, the total Black population of the eleven Southern states was approximately 10.2 million (about 51 percent of the total U.S. Black population), with 3.7 million residing in rural areas. This can be compared to a total population of the South of 62.8 million with 22.3 million (35.4) being classified as rural. The majority of the rural Black population is still concentrated in the Coast Lowlands, Coastal Plains, and Piedmont areas where the plantation as a social unit once prevailed (Map 1). The upland Appalachian area of the South, in which small commercial and subsistence farms traditionally pre-dominated, contained fewer Blacks until this century, when a small number began migrating into the area to become small farmers or to take up jobs as unskilled and semi-skilled laborers (Gastil 1975). Indeed, we find that

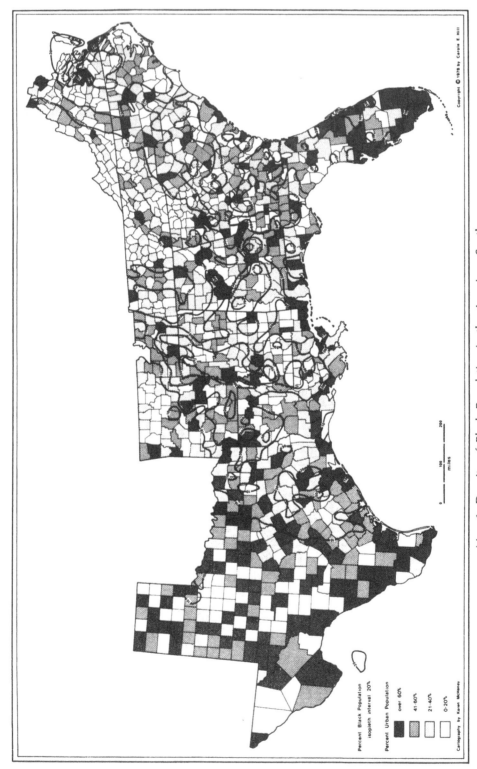

Map 1. Density of Black Population in the American South

Percent Black Population
isopleth interval 20%

Percent Urban Population

over 60%

41-60%

21-40%

0-20%

0   100   200
miles

there is an almost perfect inverse relationship between areas in the South where Blacks reside and areas where rapid economic development is taking place (Marshall 1976).

Although Blacks continued to emigrate from the South between 1960 and 1970, in most states the natural increase offset the loss of population which was due to this outmigration. Moreover, because of the outmigration and high birth rate, the age structure of the rural Black population reflects a large number of persons (approximately 50 percent) in the 0–20 year age bracket. Although it might be assumed that young men and women migrants would take their children with them, the data seems to indicate otherwise. While specific figures are not available, ethnographic studies have documented a pattern of child-sharing in black families, where older relatives keep the children of young adults who spend long periods of time away from home working. This migration has affected the household structure and reordered the social relationships in a pattern of matrilocality (Stack 1977; Jones, n.d.; Shimkin and Lowe 1972), and undoubtedly accounts in part for the age structure of the population.

Although the historical tradition of racial discrimination in the South has altered in recent decades, demographic changes have been slow, with rural areas experiencing less change than urban centers. As a result, the majority of rural Blacks today are still very poor and undereducated, and some still remain quite isolated from mainstream society. Indeed, in 1970, 52 percent of rural black families in the South earned less than $3,745 for a family of four and thus lived below the poverty level. Furthermore, the proportion of poor black to poor white families was higher in rural areas than in any other residential sector of the South. Thus the overall and predominant economic status of rural Southern blacks in 1970 was one of great poverty (median family income, $3,525). In 1970, only 3.5 percent of rural Southern black families earned $12,000 or more.

More recent statistics on the Black population (both rural and urban) of Area IV of the Public Health Service (the Southern states) indicate a substantial increase in black population in these eight Southern states (Rogers 1979). A new pattern of outmigration has emerged in the 1970s which indicates that migration has continued to decline and that the number moving to the South has increased. At the same time, the unemployment rate for Blacks increased and was about double that of Whites in 1978. The median annual income for black men ($5,370) was eroded with regard to purchasing powers, while that of women was $2,810 compared to $14,958 for the U.S. and $14,562 for the eight Southern States (Region IV). Between 1970 and 1974, the relative level of Black income did not move upward, with 34 percent of black families earning under $4,000, which is virtually the same in terms of constant dollars as in 1970. Furthermore, the overall income position of black families relative to white families declined between

1970 and 1974. Additional statistics indicate that: (1) female heads comprise a majority of all low-income families; (2) the proportion of black husband-wife families declined from 68 percent to 51 percent and the proportion of female heads increased from 28 percent to 35 percent, and (3) black female heads of families were more likely to be single or divorced in 1974 than in 1970.

In 1976, 23 percent (5.8 million) of all the persons living in poverty lived in Florida, Georgia, Tennessee, Kentucky, South Carolina, North Carolina, Alabama and Mississippi. The poverty rate for Blacks (urban and rural) was second highest in 1976 for these states, while 2.7 million (36 percent) Blacks living in poverty lived in the South. In addition, 51.6 percent of black children age 5 to 17 lived in homes below poverty level, as compared to 37.1 percent nationally (Rogers 1979). Current population reports do not break down statistics on rural and urban Blacks, so specific changes cannot be compared. In 1977, Blacks exceeded the proportions of white persons among workers in blue-collar jobs and unemployed persons (Bureau of the Census 1978). It is interesting to note that poverty in the South is basically a rural phenomenon, whereas it is a consequence of urbanism outside the region. Thus, the demographic characteristics reported in the 1970 census have demonstrated slow change among the poor and minority groups.

These changes are, in part, based on immigration patterns of the South and a redistribution of the nation's poverty population. A report on inner-regional migration of the poor states " . . . the paper's most important empirical result was to detect the southern region's [16 states plus D.C.] shift from annual net immigration of the poor between 1967 and 1977." The report further states: "Although the southern region as a whole shifted to net immigration in the 1960s, the net immigration in that decade consisted entirely of the white nonpoor population. Not until the 1970s has the South come to have net immigration of Blacks and persons below the poverty level. Clearly, the region's growing volume of net immigration in the decade is much more heterogeneous than before" (Bureau of Census 1978).

Along with poverty, the lack of education of most rural Blacks has contributed to the population's general isolation from mainstream society and medical care. Only 13.5 percent of rural Blacks over age 24 had graduated from high school in 1970, and the median number of school years completed was only slightly over seven. Since that time, the proportion of Blacks in the U.S. who have completed high school and one year of college has somewhat increased (Bureau of Census 1978). However, their lack of education as well as economic opportunity is clearly reflected in the types of occupations held by rural Blacks. We find that 63 percent of rural Black men work as operatives or laborers, while 80 percent of the women work as operatives or service and domestic workers.

The availability of health care to rural Blacks has increased in the past fifteen years. Medicaid protection is more prevalent and has allowed more rural residents the opportunity to use modern medicine, although some health practitioners question the success of Medicare and Medicaid; they feel that such programs are biased against rural areas (Wheeler 1976; Marshall 1976; Davis and Marshall 1979). Nonetheless, there appears to be an increased pattern of utilization which is due to, in addition to the Medicaid and Medicare programs, the "rural health initiative" (RHI) begun by the U.S. Public Health Service in 1975. This integrated existing programs for the purpose of improving better health care. However, health needs occur disproportionately among rural subcultures (Copp 1976) and as a consequence, health facilities must take these cultural differences into consideration when planning the delivery of health care. As rural Blacks and Whites ascend the socioeconomic ladder their basic needs will change, as well as their ideas about health and illness, and their demand for equal health care (preventive and environmental services), not just medical care. Indeed, as discussed earlier, health care cannot be discussed in our society without taking economic, social, and cultural variables into consideration.

As Seham (1973) has clearly pointed out, racism and poverty are two sides of the same coin and poor Blacks have not received the same quality of care as the more affluent Whites; he reports disparate treatment of Blacks and Whites even in the Medicaid and Medicare programs. Indeed, we find that: (1) the life expectancy of Blacks, especially black males, is still lower than for Whites; (2) obesity is more likely in black women than in white women; (3) the infant mortality rate among Blacks is 85 percent higher than among Whites; (4) fifty percent of black men between the ages of 55 and 65 have hypertension, compared to 31 percent for Whites; (5) Medicare payments are higher for Whites than Blacks; (6) health services are more extensively paid for for Whites than for Blacks; (7) white Medicaid patients receive payments for physician services that are 40 percent higher than for Blacks; and (8) there are significant numbers of the poor ineligible for Medicaid (Kennedy 1979; Wheeler 1976).

2

A Rural Community Within the Regional Context

Throughout the world, rural peoples have historically differed from urban peoples. In the United States, rural peoples have lived longer, had larger families, worked on the land, generally worn different kinds of clothing, eaten different foods, gone to different kinds of schools and churches, voted for different politicians and, most importantly for our purposes, perceived health and health care differently (Gilford, Nelson, Ingram 1981). Overall, their ideology and structures have been different from those of urban dwellers and have manifested themselves in ways that were easy to delineate.

During this century, however, people who live in rural areas are becoming difficult to distinguish from city folk. Rural people simply live farther apart, pay more for utilities such as telephones, water and electricity, and have to travel farther to stores, schools, hospitals, physicians, libraries, etc., for services. The concept of rurality is thus often reduced to a simple fact of location. Some writers, however, feel that rural culture and social structure continue to flourish and are real entities to both rural and urban dwellers (Miller and Luloff 1981; Buttel and Flinn 1975; England, et al. 1979; Fliegel 1976; Larson 1978; Lowe and Peek, 1974; Hill 1977; Miller and Crader 1979).

The empirical indicators of rural economic, social and political institutions have changed drastically. Although many Americans believe that most rural people live on farms, the 1970 census classified only 18 percent of the rural population as farmers, while 62 percent were farmers in 1920. Foresters, shopkeepers, pastors, miners, and other non-farm workers have always been a part of the rural structure, but their numbers are increasing as rural populations increase. In addition to these real changes, changes in attitudes about rural life have made clear the inadequacy of much statistical data about rural areas. Until recently rural areas have symbolized a rather "backward" way of life and, from a policy analysis standpoint, have been dismissed as residual (Gilford, et al. 1981). This attitude has resulted in statistical data which is inadequate or outmoded. Although more than half of the 39,000 local units of government in the U.S. have populations of less than 1000 and 70 percent have populations of less than 2500, relatively little is known about these governments with regard to their capacity to change and to interconnect with larger governmental units for the purpose of delivering services (Gilford, et al. 1981).

This national ignorance and neglect has, to some degree, changed during the past two decades. Changes in population trends, and in governmental policies based on the ideology of equity of services for all citizens, have called attention to rural areas. Overall, rural areas are growing faster in population than urban areas (Beale and Fuguitt 1978; Morrison and Wheeler 1976). Since 1970, the growth rate of non-metropolitan areas in the U.S. has outstripped that of metropolitan areas and the U.S. population as a whole. Indeed, the 1980 census shows that non-metropolitan counties grew in population from 1970 to 1980 by 15.4 percent, while metropolitan counties increased in population by only 9.1 percent and a 10.0 percent increase was reported for the nation as a whole (Beale 1981). The federal government has acknowledged this "back to the land" movement and in December 1979, the "small community and rural development policy" was announced. This provided incentives for small businesses to locate in rural areas. It should be pointed out, however, that this rural renaissance is extremely uneven. Some areas are growing very rapidly while more than 400 counties (predominantly minority and/or agricultural areas) are continuing to decline in population (Cornman, et al. 1981).

In addition, some studies suggest that, as mentioned earlier, there has been a convergence of demographic characteristics of rural and urban populations in the U.S. in recent years (Zuiches and Brown 1978). Rural and urban dwellers have become more similar in terms of indicators such as income, occupational status, educational attainment, household size, and labor force participation of women between 1950 and 1975. This is a result of developing industrialization in several areas, which has afforded economic opportunities especially for minority groups. Manufacturing and services are the major areas of employment of minorities in rural areas (Brown 1978). Indeed, as mentioned above, agriculture is no longer the leading industry in rural areas (Hassinger 1976).

As a consequence of these demographic trends the rural population is becoming less homogeneous as socioeconomic differences emerge. People who are moving to rural areas are bringing with them a wide range of beliefs, values and lifestyles. Although major differences between urban and rural residents remain (Larson 1978), increased heterogeneity is creating change and conflict in rural communities. Newcomers bring new ideas about how to manage resources and what innovations should be made in developing new resources. Rural dwellers are often apprehensive about growth for fear of the loss of the unique social and physical features of rural living (Doherty 1979). According to Gilford et al. (1981) many rural people wonder who will benefit from growth—the land owners, the wage-earners or the new-comers. Indeed, "growth policy is better characterized as anti-growth policy in many communities . . ." (1981:7). It appears that when change occurs, only a few groups support it. Very often, changes are implemented by immigrants who have had different life experiences and are therefore aware of the alternative resources and services that are available from the urban world.

As we shall see, the heterogeneity of the population and conflicts over resources are factors in explaining the dynamics of the development of a primary health care clinic in Coberly. Many of the traditional residents opposed the clinic—they did not feel that it was needed. The innovators who planned and implemented the clinic were considered "outsiders" and, in fact, most of the people who are working to change the community are newcomers. They are reacting to and changing a culture and social structure that can only be understood within a regional context. An understanding of both the uniqueness of the rural South and its similarities to other rural areas allows us to better analyze the cultural models and health behavior of the people in Coberly and their linkages to the medical system.

Southern Uniqueness

White Southerners, according to Killian (1970) and Reed (1972), constitute an ethnic group within the United States mainly due to their minority status with respect to the rest of the nation. These authors claim that Southerners have been discriminated against and singled out from others in the society for differential and unequal treatment due to physical and cultural characteristics, and as a consequence Southerners have created "myths" that function to maintain their distinct cultural tradition. Killian states that "no amount of elaborate pleading will overcome the arguments that may be advanced against the proposition that white Southerners are indeed a minority" (1970:4).

While white Southerners are a minority with respect to the nation as a whole, Blacks in the South, although a numerical majority in some areas, are a minority group both nationally and regionally. They have been controlled by the political and economic structures dominated by white Southerners. Because of this minority status, as we have seen in Chapter 1, they remain low on most of the indices that measure quality of life. Blacks, nonetheless, are a part of Southern society. As Myrdal (1944) stated many years ago,

"American negro culture is not something independent of general American culture. It is a distorted development, or a pathological condition, of the general American culture" (1944:928). At that time, these observations were supported in part by Dollard (1937), Davis, Gardner and Gardner (1941) and Powdermaker (1939), but they are no longer considered valid by most social scientists. Black social organization is considered as different, not deviant, from middle-class White organization.

Southern society, then, made up mostly of Blacks and Whites, has, over the years, developed a uniqueness; Whites dominate Blacks, as traditionally Southern Whites have been dominated by mainstream American society. As an adaptation to such stress, Southerners, in general, have developed a certain presentation of self that, on the one hand creates a distinctiveness in interaction and a basis for linkages and, on the other hand, forms a basis for unique cultural patterns. Again, Killian states that "the inescapable record of history and the persistence of certain cultural traits suggest that the South is truly different" (1970:9). Indeed, this theme pervades contemporary social science literature.

Tindall (1974) uses the term "ethnic" to refer to Southern distinctiveness and, interestingly, argues that the South is not dissolving into mainstream society. He says "it is not the south that has vanished, but the mainstream . . ." (1974:5). The South is a self-conscious and identifiable culture which "persists as a coherent collection of assumptions, values, traditions and commitments" (Hill 1973:18). Southern religion is a dominant factor in explaining the distinguishing characteristics of the region; religion and kinship give Southerners a set of meanings and a sense of identity that make sense of the everyday world. And these symbol systems transcend race, so that both Blacks and Whites are Southern. One author even asserts that "After centuries together, southerners, black and white, are more like one another than blacks are like Northerners" (Gastil 1975:183). Here, "symbols, beliefs and rituals are instruments used to make sense out of the social situation and to explain the conflict and contradictions creating the so-called myths of southern culture" (Hill 1977:313).

Many writers have attempted to identify the unique characteristics of Southerners. Candidates for such characteristics include localism, violence and religiosity (Reed 1972, Vandiver 1969, Hackey 1969); political conservatism (Kilpatrick 1969); antisemitism, anti-catholicism, anti-unionism (Killian 1970); poverty (Woodward 1960); racism (Phillips, 1928, 1929); laziness (Bertelson 1967); a fondness for simple-mindedness (Cash 1941); and the dominance of the plantation system (Thompson 1965). Gillin and Murphy (1951) also developed a list of traits which they felt characterized the South. All of these lists are of limited value in that they generally fail to integrate the distinct traits into a functioning dynamic system. The Gestalt of Southern culture cannot be measured by empirically counting traits.

Kinship, like religion, is an extremely important support system in the South, among both Blacks and Whites. In terms of priority of obligations, it is one's kinsmen who are of paramount importance. Instead of seeking help through outside resources, rural Southerners depend on their families to meet most of their needs, both in their daily lives and in times of crisis. There are several social mechanisms that maintain these ties, most of which are framed within a religious context. Recurrent gatherings, such as family dinners, family reunions, homecomings, decoration day and campmeetings (Neville 1975; Jones 1976; Hill 1982), function to transmit Southern culture to younger generations, as well as to solidify social obligations and a belief system, among both Blacks and Whites. Shimkin and Lowe (1971) found that the black extended family in Mississippi is a basic socio-economic mechanism in rural life there. They also found that it aids in the facilitation of migration and urbanization. Likewise, Jones (1976) demonstrated how persisting kinship ties between rural and urban areas are a resource for economic aid and a source of change. Lastly, Beaver (1986) feels that kinship networks are the basis of the social, political and economic organization of Whites in Southern Appalachia.

A strategy of Southerners, involving actual social interaction, is indirectness. Traditional Southerners generally avoid direct confrontation or situations of conflict in normal interactional settings; they prefer to handle such situations using indirect mechanisms such as "biblical dueling" and by settling disputes outside the court system, within church kinship and neighborhood networks (Greenhouse 1986), joking relationships (Peterson 1975) and religious symbolic interactions in political situations (Jones 1976). Many such interactions outside the church are based on the kind of behavior expected in church services, mainly the conversion experience and witnessing (Hill 1982). Southerners are masters at "behind-the-scenes" bargaining (i.e., Southern congressional styles), which quite often is accomplished without either party's overtly verbalizing actual goals, compromises, etc. The rules are known but unspoken. Reasonably, this strategy developed during colonial times in the Old South when a class system was emerging and Southerners, because of their European heritage, were reluctant to admit it. Consequently, the higher classes maintained contact with lower classes, giving the appearance of an egalitarian society. Indirectness, as a mode of interaction, avoids overt confrontation of social differences on the one hand and, on the other, is a manipulative device on the part of those in minority positions (whatever level).

The value placed on egalitarianism (mostly among Southern Whites) is combined with that placed on independence. Rural Southerners have resented any kind of authority; they especially rebel against governmental control, regulation and "outsiders coming into town telling them what to do." People in a rural community depend on one another through support networks

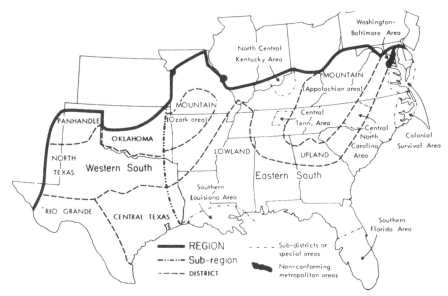

Map 2. The Subdivisions of the South. Source: Gastil (1975)

based on kinship and religious ties which, in turn, provides them with an emotionally charged security that they do not want threatened. This idea of independence is the major social control mechanism on a local level. Rural Southerners traditionally have not participated in structured politics or, for that matter, used the mainstream system on a state or national level. People most often go to the preacher or the family with their problems rather than to agencies. Many say the government has no place in their personal lives.

Indirectness and independence are cultural manifestations of a learned ability to perceive subtle features of interpersonal relationships on the one hand, and on the other hand, to maintain an expected appearance within the parameters of the majority group. These strategies have produced distinct styles of interaction (based on the Southern worldview) among both Blacks and Whites. As we shall see, these styles of interaction are present within the health system.

The Social Models of Southern Culture

Within the American South, a variety of subcultures has developed due to migration, settlement patterns, and differential adaptations to the varying environmental niches within the region (Map 2). These ethnic patterns were established early in the history of the South and have remained much the same in rural areas. Only recently have urban areas experienced the immigration of large numbers of ethnic groups (Hill 1980).

During the 17th and 18th centuries, the region was settled mostly by the British (concentrated in Virginia and the coastal regions of North and South Carolina), and to a lesser extent by the Spanish (Florida and Texas) and the French (Coastal region of the Gulf of Mexico). It was the British, however, who adapted to frontier life and, along with American Indians and Blacks, became the receiving end for further migrations. A majority of these English people were elite and, according to Gastil, "Instead of being a 'new start' in a new world, the elite of the 17th and 18th century South saw themselves as recreating the old world, often as recreating an old world that in fact had already ceased to exist" (1975:177). In 1790, 81.3 percent of the White population of the South was English, Scottish and Scotch-Irish. In the 18th century, Scotch-Irish and Germans migrated from Pennsylvania to the valleys of Virginia and into the southern Piedmont. They were joined by Scottish-Highlanders and Scotch-Irish who emigrated from Scotland and Ireland, entering the country through the ports of Charleston and Wilmington. The Scotch-Irish were the largest group to move south, most being Presbyterians.

The second largest group was the Germans, mostly Protestants from Austria and the Rhine region, and, unlike the former group, they remained isolated, having little to do with politics, slavery or the plantation system. Consequently, they had little influence on basic Southern social patterns. It was the English, Scots (lowlanders and highlanders) and Scotch-Irish who formed the basis of the social and cultural patterns of the American South. After 1850, any significant number of foreign-born Whites who immigrated to the region settled on the fringes (Gastil 1975).

These migrants all brought with them their own forms of religious observance, and in order to understand the nature of rurality, it is imperative to examine the impact religion has had on this form of life. Indeed, the most outstanding characteristic of white Protestantism in American is its ruralism (Anderson 1970). Most of the early Protestant churches developed in rural areas, with two-thirds of all white Protestants living in localities of under 100,000 people. Anderson feels that within the first generation, the settlers and immigrants from Europe turned from their origins to religion as a basis for identity, with the church being the center for rural ethnic group life. The English were Episcopal (Anglican) and Congregational, the Scottish were Presbyterians, and the Germans were Lutherans.

The extensive spread of Methodists and Baptists, who won converts from all the ethnic groups in the region, occurred relatively late in the 19th century. The power base for Baptists was in the North, with only 25 Baptist churches found in the South in 1750. A century later, their churches remained few in various subareas of the South (tidewater regions), a pattern that remains today; most Baptist churches are still concentrated within the interior of the region. Likewise, the Methodists were late arrivals and, from a point of concentration in the Northeast, initially began to move westerly with circuit riders rather than southerly, following the roads that opened up on the frontier (Gaustod 1972). At present, however, the Methodist Church is surpassed in numbers only by Baptists in the South. Thus, a majority of Blacks and Whites now are fundamentalist Protestants and are either Methodists or Baptists.

The other major ethnic group to come to the South was Blacks. The first Blacks came from West Africa involuntarily, as slaves to work on the plantations. Their descendants have lived to contemporary times under the edifice of and belief in racism. The class structure of the rural regions of the South can still be described as being controlled by Whites in terms of power and authority, even though in many areas, Blacks are in the majority. Slavery was originally justified as a good and positive force and as part of the normal order of society. This "Doctrine of White Supremacy," combined with a desire for land (and thus power), underwrote the importance of slaves for labor needs on the plantation. Most slaves were brought into the South in the late 1700s and early 1800s; their numbers then began to increase. For example, in 1820 there were 1,643,000 Blacks; in 1860 there were 4,097,000. Also in 1860, there were about 900 plantations of 1000 or more acres in the state in which Coberly is located (Simkins 1963). There were also a few free Blacks in the region who either farmed or worked in the towns.

After the Civil War, many Blacks moved North, and with the coming of industrialization in the early part of the 20th century, both Blacks and Whites migrated to Northern cities or to large towns and cities in the South. The Blacks who remained in rural areas continued to live with racism, and as we shall see, are today generally poorer than the Whites. They have only recently been given an opportunity for mobility in the caste-like system that has pervaded the rural South.

So, early on, the South stabilized with a predominate make-up of two ethnic groups—Blacks and Whites—with the Whites dominating and defining the social and political system. Black inequality underpinned relationships and, until recently, remained the accepted and expected basis for public and private decision-making. As a consequence, Blacks developed a social structure and culture that was an adaptation to its position in a society whose political economy was dominated by Whites. There was very little new immigration after the Civil War; in fact, the South lost population to the rest of the nation. It thus stabilized as a relatively Old American White society that turned inward and, like its Blacks, developed a structure and culture to adapt to their position in American society. Many years ago Odum (1936) observed that the South (exclusive of Blacks) was the most

"American" of all regions. Indeed, in many ways it crystallized into the rather static ideal type that the Protestants who settled the area had visualized.

From this base, the South developed "several versions of Southern culture in terms of somewhat contrasting models" (Pearsall 1966:128). After pointing out that the South has never been, and is not now, homogenous in terms of culture and structure, she delineates two models, the "Frontier" and the "Plantation." The former encompasses Appalachian areas, while the latter developed in the coastal plain and Piedmont subregions. Although they practically overlap in time and space, as models they are distinguishable and provide guidelines for delineating different lifestyles. The frontier model denotes what is basically a "mountain" way of life lived, until recently, in isolated villages whose social organization is based on kinship ties. Here people have valued independence and egalitarianism and, until external developmental stresses appear (such as coal mining and lumbering), have remained relatively unchanged.

The plantation model was limited both geographically and socially, being built mostly upon the cotton and rice economy. It is from this model that the stereotypes of Southern society, its men and women, have developed. Ironically, in terms of numbers, this model was in the minority, but it was very powerful. It was in plantation areas that Blacks were concentrated (and continue to be, at least rural Blacks). According to Rubin (1951), the major themes in the plantation model are: (1) mastery of the land (power rests in control of the land); (2) conformity with the word of God (fundamentalist Protestantism in which upper-class Whites interpreted Calvinism to prove God's favor symbolized by material possessions; religious opposition to worldly pleasures); (3) ideal stratification of humankind (race-caste based on White supremacy).

The majority of Southerners were yeoman farmers, the "plain folk of the old South" (Owsley 1949). This model refers to the subsistence farmers and townspeople who were not as wealthy as the plantation owners and who did not really participate extensively in the plantation system. It overlaps spatially and chronologically with the frontier model, although most "plain folk" (both Black and White) did not live in the mountains. They were a target for the Baptist and Methodist evangelists (Bruce 1974). As they prospered, a few mixed the frontier model with the plantation model. Most, however, remained poor and "lived intimately with each other in a small and personal world. Neighbors were our kind of folks, and the other subgroups were ours, too—'our negroes,' 'our white folks,' 'our workers' and even 'our poor whites'" (Pearsall 1966:138). This folk model has given way somewhat to more impersonal relations and a more open worldview in some rural areas, especially the areas where "outsiders" have moved. It remains, however, a strong force in the social and cultural world of many rural Southerners. A majority still "live concretely in terms of particular places and people and the repetitiveness of the past in the present" (Pearsall 1966:141).

The heirs to these traditions are the indigenous Southerners who live in rural areas and small towns, and who provide a key to understanding continuity and change in the rural South. The people of Coberly participate in these cultural, social and ecological models which give us a background against which we can better understand the heterogeneity of their health behavior and beliefs; how they are similar to and different from one another, and how they differentially link to the medical system that is superimposed on their health systems.

Cober County:
Levels of Organization and Resources

Cober County combines the plantation and folk traditions with a social structure based on racial segregation and an economic structure similar to that of poor yeoman farmers. It is located 50 miles from the state capital, Magnolia, and 15 miles from the city of Bulla. A major north-south highway runs through the county and, along with buslines and country roads, connects the county seat, Coberly, with the outside world. There are no active railroad stations. The average temperature for the year is 62.9 degrees F (45.8 in winter and 79.1 in summer), and the average annual rainfall is 5.1 inches.

A drive through the county reveals the calmness of rolling hills; a few large farms have herds of cattle and fields with small lakes. Pecan orchards interrupt open pastures dotted with horses. The fields are green most of the year with crops. Houses vary from a few large 19th-century structures to the modest frame houses in which most Blacks and Whites live.

Five towns are located in the county, the largest being Coberly with a population of 995. The nearest town to Coberly, Milbyville, with 317 people, is named for the Primitive Baptist Church, and was established in 1866. In the 19th century it had a hotel, 3 cotton gins, a grist mill, a fertilizer plant, a grain elevator and a canning plant, but now it has only a few stores and a gas station. Nevertheless, its citizens had it entered on the National Register of Historic Places. Holladay, a town of 303 people, grew up around a railway stop. Today most of its people work outside the town or make a living in the pecan industry. Holladay has seven churches. The two additional towns in the county, Angleton (population 379) and Oliverville (population 250) have changed little over the years, with most activity centering around the cotton economy and/or the railroad. Oliverville was once a stopping point on the New York to New Orleans Rail Line. The streets of Oliverville were paved in 1961 and city water service began in 1966.

Cober County came into being in 1822 with land acquired from local Indians via a treaty between them and the state. Commissions were appointed and the courthouse square was set up in the county seat. The first permanent courthouse was built in 1826-27, and in 1895, the present courthouse was constructed in Coberly. Religion was important to the founders, so the churches were, as they still are, a focal point for linkages and identity in the community. The first churches built were Baptist and Methodist. As in most of the rural South, circuit riders came to preach at monthly intervals. Campgrounds were established in the early 1800s near a spring. As was typical of the era, Blacks and Whites used the same churches but the times of their services were different. The Methodists would allow Blacks to sit in galleries during the Whites' services.

In the early 1800s, there were two separate schools, one for girls and another for boys. Later, however, an academy was established (1889) with 58 students. In 1891, three students graduated from the academy, and in 1902, it was deeded to the Methodist Church. In 1912, it was deeded to the county Board of Trustees and became the county high school. The enrollment was 117 in 1917. Blacks attended another school until the schools were consolidated in 1969. Today, both Blacks and Whites attend the only high school in the county. Now there is also a first grade center for kindergarten through first grade, a primary school for kindergarten through second grade, an elementary school for grades three through six, and a junior high for grades seven through nine. In addition, there has been a church-sponsored children's home in the county since 1940.

Since its formation, the size of the county has been reduced by the formation of three other counties from its original area. This division of Cober County occurred at different times during a span of almost a hundred years. Perhaps the most significant loss caused by this reduction in size was the annexation of two cities to the newly founded counties. There are no city-sized towns in Cober County today. The lack of the resources that cities offer has affected the tax base of the county and has diminished its attractiveness as a location for business and industry. Currently, 9,000 people live in Cober County, but most wage-earners must go outside the county to work.

Farming and ties to the land were important to the early inhabitants. In the first half of the nineteenth century, cotton, rice, wheat and corn were grown on large farms. The single large plantation in the county was owned by C. Coberly. Coberly owned a number of slaves, a large lumber mill and a furniture factory. He opened the first circular saw mill in the area, and designed a wooden screw cotton press which was widely used for baling cotton.

Although plantations like Coberly's were relatively common in this part of the state, most people were yeoman farmers. In the last half of the nineteenth century cotton declined in importance and diversification of crops became a necessity for these farmers. Crops such as soybeans, peaches, pimentos (the chief cash crop in the 1950s) and pecans were grown. Eventually, these began to decline and poultry production began to become important for farm incomes. Historically, small business enterprises such as grist mills, cotton gins, blacksmith shops, stores, hotels, and family pottery operations were also scattered among the towns and villages of Cober County. There was still at least one blacksmith shop remaining in the county during the 1940s, a water-powered grist mill operated until 1950, and a cotton gin was in operation as late as the 1970s. Agriculture and small business prevail today, although light industries such as food processing, apparel-making and lumber operations have become the principal employment opportunities for the people of Cober County.

The major industries in the county—agriculture, construction, light manufacturing—employ most of the residents. A large percentage, however, travel outside the county for work, mostly to neighboring counties, and a few drive to Magnolia. The latter category consists generally of immigrants and not of indigenous inhabitants. In 1980, a total of 720 people were employed by industry in the county (turkey and pecan processing). An average of 375 worked in manufacturing (apparel and other textile products), 138 in contract construction, 57 in retail trade, 67 in services, and an average of 60 each in finance, insurance, and real estate. Fewer than 20 people work in the wholesale trade or transportation and other public utilities (see Table 10).

The majority of the people are poor (Black and White) with 27 percent of the county's population below the poverty level. At least 40 percent of persons over 65 are below the poverty level. The median household income is $6,652, with 12 percent of the population making over $15,000. The unemployment rate is about nine percent, and a large number of people are dependent on government subsidies. In 1978, over 4 percent of the households received Aid to Families with Dependent Children (AFDC), 6.3 percent of the households received Food Stamps, 11 percent received Medicaid, and 20 percent received Social Security. In 1980 the county received a total of $10,952 in federal grants and funds.

These statistics are indicative of the economic level of the county and also of its age structure. Twenty-five percent of the population is between the ages of 1 and 14 years, while 10 percent is between 15 and 19 years, 32 percent is between 20 and 44 years and 13 percent is over 65 years of age. Within the past decade, the percentage of the population over 65 has decreased while the middle-range ages are increasing, reflecting immigration trends into the county. The average Medicaid reimbursement per recipient

TABLE 10
Cober County Employment (1980)

County Employment Summary Industries	Firms	Total	Male	Female
20 Food	3	106	46	60
21 Tobacco	0			
22 Textile	0			
23 Apparel	1	220	40	180
24 Lumber	0			
25 Furniture	1	4	4	0
26 Paper	0			
27 Printing	0			
28 Chemicals	1	3	2	1
29 Petroleum refining	0			
30 Rubber/Plastic	0			
31 Leather	0			
32 Stone/Clay/Glass	0			
33 Primary metal	0			
34 Fabricated metal	1	3	3	0
35 Non-electrical machinery	0			
36 Electrical machinery	0			
37 Transportation equipment	0			
38 Instruments	0			
39 Miscellaneous manufacturing	0			
Manufacturing	7	336	95	241
Non-manufacturing	62	3,761	NA	NA
Total	69	4,097	NA	NA

Source: Regional Health Systems Agency, Inc., Statistical Profile, 1980.

is $500.00 and the average Medicare reimbursement per enrollee is $275.00. The 13 percent of people over 65 years old is significantly higher than that in the state as a whole (9 percent). In addition, the number of years of education completed is below the state average. The people of Cober County have a median of 8.8 years of schooling completed, with a six percent dropout rate. The median for the state is 11 years, with a dropout rate of five percent.

The County has a Commission-type government, with a Mayor, City Manager and Council located in the county seat of Coberly. There are six full-time policemen and no firemen. However, 35 people have volunteered as firemen in case of an emergency. The county does not provide a garbage service, although the city of Coberly does. Coberly is also where the post office (established in 1824) and public library are found. Only one bank is located in Cober County, with assets of approximately 11 million dollars. Recently the Chamber of Commerce has become active in economic development activities by supporting the location of small industries in the area.

Recreational facilities for the people of Cober County include 10 tennis courts, 2 golf courses, 4 swimming pools and 1 country club; there are no parks. The private country club, established in 1968, currently has 65 members. There are 3 civic clubs in the county. The Lion's Club was chartered in 1946 and is very active in civic activities. The American Legion began in 1959 and has about 175 members. There are also 2 active Masonic Lodges in the county. The 3 restaurants in the county are all located in Coberly; there are no hotels or motels.

There are 30 Protestant churches in the county, 10 of which are found in Coberly. They are all Baptist, Methodist or Holiness. The nearest Roman Catholic Church is 12 miles away in the area's largest town, Bellah. The nearest Jewish Synagogue is located 50 miles away in the state's largest city, Magnolia.

Health in Cober County

A variety of factors in Cober County have affected the general health status of its population. The small size of the county, its rural status, and low county revenues have combined to limit the delivery of health services within the county. The first public health nurse began practicing there in 1941 and the Cober County Health Department was established in 1945. The health department office was located in a former service station and nutshop near Coberly. The nurse handled mainly school immunizations and home visits. She left in 1950 and the second public health nurse stayed until 1972. In 1954, the department moved to its present building in Coberly.

Today, the Cober County Health Department's functions are numerous, and until recently have been expanded to include, on paper at least: immunizations, investigations and follow-ups on communicable diseases; case-finding and treatment of tuberculosis and venereal diseases; pre-natal and post-partum care; family planning clinics and counseling; well-baby clinics; services for the chronically ill and geriatrics; drug-dependence, alcoholism, mental health and mental retardation cases; crippled children and school health problems; vision and hearing screening tests; environmental health inspections and protection of all water supplies; insect and rodent control; food and milk sanitation; sewage and solid waste disposal services; any problem that would create a health hazard (Table 11). In reality, the services performed at the time of study were fewer than these stated functions; they included no mental health services or services to the elderly. The daily schedule mostly involves family planning, prenatal care, and giving shots. The health department has a weak linkage to the newly established primary health care clinic in Coberly.

Other health services that have linked to the medical system in the county have included a private physician resident in the county and, until the 1960s, lay midwives. The county has had a total of 35 physicians since its founding, and with the exception of the period between 1972 and 1981,

TABLE 11
Cober County Public Health Department Services and
Number of Individuals Served (1980)

Clinic	Number Reached	Frequency	Staff
WIC	168	Every 6 months	R.N.
Cancer screening	5	Monthly	R.N.
EPSDT	48	Weekly	R.N.
Family planning	93	Monthly	Dr. Wright
Prenatal clinic	17	Monthly	R.N.
General health clinic		Weekly	R.N.
Well baby/Child	117		R.N.
Vision/Hearing/Dental	65		R.N.
Immunizations	1,082		R.N.
Anemia	9		R.N.
Diabetes	8		R.N.
Hypertension	160		R.N.
Parasites	7		R.N.
Venereal disease	7		R.N.
Crippled children	30		R.N.
Tuberculosis	114		R.N.

Source: Regional Health Systems Agency, Inc., Statistical Profile, 1980.

one has practiced in the county since its formation. The newly constructed primary health care clinic brought the first physician to the county after the nine-year period (1972–81) with no physician. There are no dentists, hospitals, or emergency services in the county. If an emergency occurs, an ambulance must come from a hospital in a neighboring county, or a police car is used to take the person to the nearest hospital. One pharmacy in Coberly serves the people of the entire county.

The regional psychiatric hospital is located almost 100 miles from the county. The county average for resident in-patient psychiatric care per 10,000 population is 25, higher than the regional or state rate. There is a mental health clinic in Bellah, 11 miles from Coberly, that averages treating 3.9 out-patients per 10,000 population from Cober County, significantly lower than the regional (65.2) or state (64.3) rate. In addition, a nursing home with 50 licensed beds is located in the county.

The Cober County Department of Family and Children Services (originally the Welfare Department) was begun in 1937 for the purpose of helping indigents. The Department soon added aid to dependent children and their parents, the disabled and the blind. These services were later extended to include adoption services and services to abused and neglected children. The department provides help with Food Stamps, referrals to Vocational Rehabilitation, certification for the cancer program, medical and surgical help, and prosthesis. According to the area planning commission, about 19 percent of the population uses Medicaid and/or Medicare, 31 percent is considered indigent and 50 percent use private insurance.

The regional planning commission developed a senior citizens' center in the county in 1980 that was operational until 1983. Located in Coberly, it served about 75 people a month, 3 of whom were above the poverty line. The principal function of the center was to serve meals to the participants, most being female and Black. The meals were delivered to the center in hot boxes from Magnolia (60 miles away). The elderly were picked up throughout the county in the center's van in late morning and returned home in early afternoon. Additional functions of the center were to educate the participants about nutrition, to discuss mental health problems, and to expand their awareness. It is estimated by the planning commission that 629 elderly persons need this service. A limited home health care program was also begun to provide services to a few people in the county. These services operated out of a county hospital and upon physician's orders, skilled nursing care, physical therapy, speech therapy, and nutrition counseling were provided. Because of cutbacks in funding on the national level for such programs, they no longer exist in the county.

Indicators of the health status of the people of Cober County are not significantly different from state statistics. The average life expectancy for Whites is 72.6 years and 61 years for Blacks. The number of live births per 1000 population is 17.4, higher than the state rate (15.6), although interestingly, the Black birth rate is 15 per 1000 as compared to 23 per 1000 for the state, while the White birth rate in Cober county is 19 per 1000 as compared to 13.5 per 1000 for the state. A majority of the births in the county are to teenage women, with Blacks averaging 181 per 1000 (state 265 per 1000) and Whites averaging 163 per 1000 (state 135 per 1000). Thus, the Black teenage pregnancy rate is lower in Cober County than state-wide. However, Blacks' infant death rate (under one year) is much higher—70 per 1000 as compared to 22 for the state—and neo-natal deaths (under 28 days) are 46.5 per 1000 and 69 per 1000 respectively, while the infant death rate is 0 for Whites.

The leading causes of death in Cober county are shown in Table 12. The four leading causes of death among Blacks and Whites in 1979 were heart disease, cerebrovascular disease, cancer and cirrhosis of the liver. In 1984 however, when statistics are broken down by race, differences emerge between the races especially in areas of accidents, mental disorders and cirrhosis of the liver. Granted these are small numbers but the patterns they represent are consistent for the past two decades. Cancer is the leading cause of morbidity, with gonorrhea reported second. Other indicators of health status for the county include a rather high arrest rate for driving under the influence (26 per 1000), a low rate for narcotic drug arrests (2.5 per 1000), a moderate number of delinquency cases (6.8 per 1000) and no reported cases of child abuse.

TABLE 12
Mortality Rates in Cober County 1976, 1984 per 100 Population

Major Causes of Death	1976		1984			
	(Black/White)	(rate)	White	(rate)	Black	(rate)
Disease of the circulatory system	28	(372.4)	39	(512.0)	11	(493.7)
Malignant neoplasms	14	(186.2)	7	(91.9)	2	(89.8)
Cerebrovascular disease	16	(212.8)	14	(183.8)	4	(179.5)
Injury and poisoning	--	--	11	(144.4)	2	(89.0)
Disease of the respiratory system	1	(13.3)	6	(78.8)	0	(0)
Suicides	2	(26.6)	2	(26.3)	0	(0)
Homocides	13	(15.6)	2	(26.3)	0	(0)
Mental disorders	--	--	1	(13.1)	2	(89.8)
Diabetes mellitus	2	(26.6)	1	(13.1)	0	(0)
Cirrhosis of liver	3	(39.9)	1	(13.1)	2	(89.8)
Infectious and parasitic disease	--	--	0	(0)	1	(44.9)

Source: Regional Health Systems Agency, Inc., Statistical Profile, 1980; and
Georgia Division of Epidemiology, Department of Human Resources, 1984.

Obviously, a cause of most of the diseases discussed above is behavior or "lifestyle." This fact is a stressor on the biomedical approach to health and the system it organizes in rural areas. Before exploring how the system responds to these health problems, and how the people use their social/ cultural systems to adjust to their problems, let us look at the people of Coberly.

The People of Coberly

Coberly is a typical rural Southern town whose people, for the most part, conform to the traditional plantation and folk model in Southern society. In 1980, the population of the community was 995 people, an increase over the 1970 population of 776. Of these people, 626 are White (53 percent) and 468 are Black (47 percent), with 5 Hispanics and 1 Asian. Following the normal housing patterns in the rural South, Blacks live in separate sections of town from Whites, with some integration occurring in transitional areas. Altogether the households in the town number 296.

Indeed, by including social and economic characteristics with the cultural system in this rural community, we have a picture of a rather typical traditional, rural, Southern town, although it is not as isolated as some communities in the region. The people can be divided into various classes or strata and such categorization can prove useful in explaining health beliefs and behavior. The people of Coberly are aware of their various statuses and the constraints placed on them. They are, nonetheless, decision makers and attempt to control the things which they feel they can control.

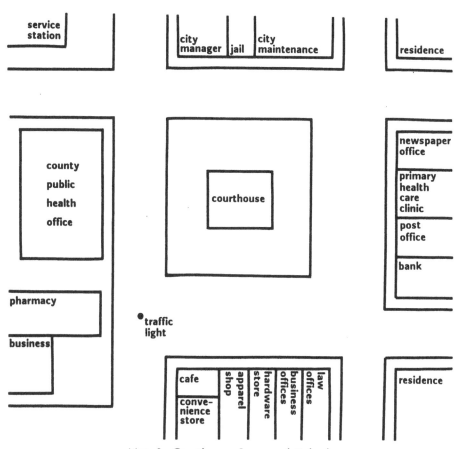

Map 3. Courthouse Square of Coberly

As we shall see, certain aspects of their health behavior are completely controlled by them. The kind of control however, varies with income and ethnicity.

The threads that hold the community together are family and neighborhood relationships and a sense of geographical boundary (Map 3). Both provide a security and identity for the people. Geographical bonding begins cognitively with a person's house and its relationship to the town square.

The center of town is a main business area with a courthouse square. Across the street to the east are the city and county services, such as the jail and the city maintenance and city manager's offices. On the west side of the courthouse are shops and business offices and until recently (1984), the most popular cafe in the county was located here. Most of the white collar workers lunched, conducted business or met friends in the cafe. It was here that many of the informal linkages between the state, regional and local levels were created and maintained. At the present time, these mediations take place in a much larger town outside the county.

The county public health clinic and pharmacy lie to the south of the courthouse and the newly constructed primary health care clinic, along with the post office, bank and newspaper office, are directly to the west of the courthouse. Parking is available on three sides of the courthouse. On a typical day, one can always find several empty spaces. The rhythm of activity is slow; one rarely observes a crowd (with the exception of special activities in the courthouse). Very few people are in the stores at any one time and it is rare to pass people while walking on the streets. Because very few people come to town, it can be assumed that the town is dying. The latter is a false assumption, as we shall discuss later. When compared to those in an urban center, however, the people appear slow, unhurried and unconcerned about the outside world.

Residential houses are very near the square, as shown in Map 3. These are white areas with a number of large old houses, some of which have been renovated. Most of the houses are poorly kept up and are rather run down. Older white people live in most of these homes; many are moderately furnished. In these areas near the square, most people live on a subsistence income, mostly from Social Security supplemented by wages from odd jobs, and of the people interviewed in this area, the average income was just over $5,000.

Most of these people are old-time residents of the town and take pride in their community. Many take walks every day after supper around part of the square or the neighborhood. Their sons and daughters mostly live in another town or another county. They look forward to Sundays or special occasions when the family will get together. Some of these people are members of the Methodist church, others are Baptists, and still others are Holiness. They talk about their families a lot and take pride in the historical foundation of their community and their heritage. Most had been farmers or worked for someone who owned a farm. Now, they sit and watch their community change and talk about "those outsiders" who change everything. These attitudes are important in the following chapter as I discuss the mechanisms for change in the health care delivery system in Coberly.

As we move northward, the neighborhood slowly becomes black, with some white families living side by side with Blacks. They are all poor. Farther away from the square, the residents are all black. At the outer limits of the town in this direction is the newest of the two black neighborhoods in the community. The social patterns here are not integrated as in the other black neighborhood, although we observed some visiting patterns. The houses are all wooden, most are unpainted, and all have some sort of garden. Indeed, two residents told me that if it were not for the garden, they would not be able to eat properly. The furnishings in these houses are often meager, with old repaired and make-shift furniture. There are always places to sit, most frequently on the front porch. Only one house in this area has an air conditioner.

The houses here are scattered (from 500 yards to 1/2 mile apart) and the income varied. Because this is a new black area of Coberly, there are fewer kinship ties beyond the household, making the neighborhood less cohesive and homogeneous than the older black neighborhood. Most of these people's ties are found across town. One household here is headed by a 43-year-old woman named Elsie who works five days a week to "keep up" her four sons, ages 8 to 23 years old. She does not know her immediate neighbor very well and would have to call on one three houses away if she needed help. Her closest neighbors to the south are an elderly couple who complain about the "goings on" in her house: "All that drinking and who knows what else." They often call the police to report loud noises from Elsie's house.

Two generations live in nearly all of the households (mostly with a woman as head of household) in this area, with the one exception of a middle-aged couple, whose children have moved away. A few of these people do not know the names of their neighbors. Furthermore, a majority of them do not attend church regularly although they all feel that belief in Jesus is essential for a good life.

Beginning from the square again, we move to the west where we find, for the most part, a middle-class neighborhood with well-kept, well-furnished houses with the yards properly manicured by a gardener. About fifty percent of these houses are brick and were constructed within the past 30 years. The remaining ones are older wood frames, painted with green shingles, surrounded by large trees. This is the wealthiest neighborhood within the town limits. The incomes vary, although everyone can be classified as middle-class. Many are professionals who look to the outside for economic support and send their children to college. Most of these houses have rather expensive furnishings, and many of their residents have maids or cleaning women who come at least once a week.

None of these households have over two generations living together and many are occupied by couples whose children have moved out—sometimes down the street or across town "on the eastside." There is a sense of community in this area, the structure of which is held together by family and kinship, religion and voluntary organizations. The important institutions are the church and the civic organizations. A large white Methodist church is located on the east boundary of this neighborhood. A majority of the people attend every Sunday and support its activities, while a few attend the Baptist church. The men who live in this area are the leaders in the Lion's Club and the American Legion and, to a lesser extent, the Masonic

Lodge. They basically dominate the Chamber of Commerce and have informal linkages to the power structure of the town, county and state. The women are active not only in church activities, but also in the Garden Club. Daily activities of the men involve working during the week, attending civic meetings at night or on weekends, maintaining the house and yard (if there isn't a gardener), sometimes participating in community organized sports and attending church on Sundays. Women's activities are based on their concept of a wife/mother; i.e., attending to household chores, cooking, taking care of the children, going shopping and participating in community organizations, most of which are church based. On weekends, friends and families will visit and sometimes, families will drive into Magnolia or Bellah for dinner or entertainment (movie, play, baseball game, etc.). Unlike in other neighborhoods, very little activity can be observed here during the day.

These men and women have a sense of history that ties them to their community and to their past. This continuity with the past is the basis for their sense of the future and the changes taking place in the community. In fact, a majority of the "newcomers" who live in the community choose this area to live in. While some settle just south of the square, most feel more comfortable with people who are similar socially and culturally. The "newcomers" are often retired professional people or young middle-class families who have chosen to live in a rural area. They are more readily accepted by the people in this neighborhood who take pride in their community.

In this area, a majority of the residents, like Whites in other areas, feel that religion is an important part of their lives. They believe in the Bible and, for the most part, are fundamentalists in their interpretation of its meaning. The bases of values and morals are the teachings of the Bible and the preaching of their pastor. The messages they receive from the church reinforce their traditional beliefs and tell them that their place in the community is proper. The meaning they derive from these symbols creates a worldview that most of these people are satisfied with in their everyday lives. These religious symbols provide a basis for their concepts of the family (the basic social unit) and health, as we shall see in subsequent chapters. This neighborhood was the least receptive to being observed and interviewed.

Returning to the square and moving south past the senior citizens' center, we first encounter a white neighborhood, with wooden houses that are not as well cared for as in the other white neighborhoods in the town. A few have old junk cars in the front yard and often several older automobiles surround the house in yards that are generally grown up. There are two apartment buildings in this area, just behind the businesses that face the main highway through town. It is in this area that we find the agricultural extension agency and the public health clinic. The incomes of the people in this neighborhood are low and most can be classified as "working class." The furnishings in their houses are adequate but the houses are not elaborately decorated. More women who live in this neighborhood hold jobs and their outside activities are mostly limited to the church and family. They have to rely on extended families and friends to help them with daily activities such as taking care of children, shopping and cooking. The men attend church less frequently and often "go off with the boys" to drink or play pool. They have less sense of community than other Whites or the Blacks.

As we move farther south, we find some light industry and some businesses such as a beer store, service station and fast food market. (Generally the people become poorer the farther away the neighborhood is from the square.) Just past the high school begins the other black neighborhood in Coberly which, because of its history of being closely integrated, I will describe in some detail.

A two-lane road runs through the middle of the neighborhood. Fewer than a half-dozen short roads run perpendicular to this highway; none of them crosses it. Some are paved while some remain dirt. Most of the houses face these roads or the highway. A few are tucked back into less accessible places off the roads. Houses of different sizes, styles, ages, and building materials are juxtaposed, with a few trailers mixed in. They sit on lots of various sizes, and some have enough acreage around them for the small-scale farming that is done. Others have neat patches of mixed vegetable and flower gardens during the spring and summer. There are grassy lawns, but there are also dirt yards of the type that is common in rural regions of the South. Most of the area is shaded by trees. Although there are a few slightly run-down houses in the neighborhood, the area is reasonably neat and well-kept. No trash piles, loose-lying junk, or evidence of vandalism or extreme property neglect detract from its appearance. The interiors of the homes where we interviewed were clean and neat, although some had more elaborate furnishings than others. There are no businesses in the neighborhood except for a former general store that is now a small billiard room with three or four playing tables; the proprietor sells cold drinks and snack foods. A church is located at the edge of the neighborhood.

The income spread of the sample households in our survey—from $1,000 to $15,000 with most between $6,000 to $8,000—is related to the number of wage earners and the sources of income. At the time of my interviews, the wage earners in four of the homes were retired or semi-retired. Of the two adults in another household, one was on disability payments and the other was unable to work because of serious health problems. This group formed the smallest income category. All of the other households in the sample (74 percent) had at least one wage earner with a full-time job or occupation. These jobs included cleaning jobs, maintenance work, construction work, cook for a business or institution, school bus driver, caretaker of children or retarded adults, elementary school teachers, mechanic, body and fender repair, and various production line jobs in a textile mill or small clothing manufacturing plant. Aside from the disabled individual, no one said he or she received public assistance payments.

As in all the other neighborhoods, people of all ages were observed and interviewed here. The oldest interviewed was ninety-eight. A few households had three generations living together. The sizes of the households ranged from one to eleven members, with an average of 3.9. The usual residence pattern here is for young, teenaged, or grown children to live with their parents. In a few cases, grandchildren live with one or more grandparents. In these instances, the grandchildren are teenagers or adults. It is not uncommon for married children to live on the same street as their parents.

During the interviews, we observed a variety of structural arrangements in the households; the nuclear family arrangement is uncommon. For example, an older retired couple had their foster daughter and her two young children living with them. They referred to her as their daughter at first. However, when we came to the pre-natal section of the interview schedule, they said she was their adopted daughter and that they had not had children themselves. After that, they said that they had never actually adopted her. Because of this, her mother was able to come and take her away from them once. The mother, who lived in Magnolia at the time, abused the girl emotionally and physically. She ran away from her mother and somehow made her way back to this couple. The girl later got married and moved to Texas. Recently, she separated from her husband and came back to Coberly with her children to live with her "parents." There had also been an elderly brother of one of them living there until recently when he was taken to a nursing home because he became too ill to be cared for at home. Later, there was a black wreath on their door; the brother had died. The couple also "keeps an eye out" for an elderly, deaf cousin who lives across the street. His children all live out of state. They take him to his doctor for frequent checkups or when he is sick, and do other errands for him.

Family and neighborhood support these people. For example, when a man in his nineties had to have his leg amputated his children got together and decided that someone had to move in to care for him, since he is a widower. It was agreed that a daughter, who is divorced with no children at home, would quit her job and care for him. The other children and some grandchildren provide them with financial support. The support provided by the family is not purely economic, moreover. All of the houses on the short road where the man lives belong to his daughters and their husbands, and one of his granddaughters lives next door to him with her husband and two children. Everyone pitches in to share yard work and cleaning and maintenance chores for the man and his daughter. Other family members, who do not live on the same road, come often to visit and bring them things. From conversations at different times with several of the family members, it became evident that they are extremely proud of him for the kind of father and husband he has been over the years. They do not think of him as a drain on family resources or a burden. According to them, he is an asset to the family that they are lucky to have. The family collectively gives economic, social, emotional, and caretaking support to him.

Residents who leave the neighborhood often feel responsibility for their kinspeople or fictive kinspeople. For example, a man in his seventies lives alone because his wife is dead and all of his children live in Ohio or Michigan now. The children have tried to persuade him to come live with one of them, but he doesn't want to leave his home or give up his independence. Other family members who live in the neighborhood, along with his neighbors, watch for him every day. Since he is always active, if he's not seen working in his field behind the house or tinkering around the shed in his yard, someone goes over to check on him. When he is sick or has an accident, one of the neighbors, a family member, or his doctor calls his children, who keep in contact regularly in any case. If the situation (which is evaluated by the doctor) is serious enough, one of the children comes and gets him and takes him back to live with him, or her while he is being treated and is recovering. Then when he is well again, one of them brings him back home. The son, who told of several such episodes, did so matter-of-factly. Although other family members in the neighborhood could have cared for the man, his children want the responsibility of caring for him when he is incapacitated. It is obvious that the people in this neighborhood, the oldest area in the town, have strong ties and feel as though this area is "their community." These ties and feelings do not extend to the other black neighborhood previously described; it is referred to as "the people from the other side of town," and derogatory statements such as "they drink too much" or "the kids do dope" or "those folks carry on" are made about it.

There is a sense of shared history and values in this neighborhood. Most people attend church regularly and feel that religion is very important in their lives. Next to the family, the church is their most important support system. The activities of the church create a social and symbolic system that, as we shall see, functions as a resource for their survival. People talk about their trust in God and, as we shall discuss in a subsequent chapter, their religious beliefs are inextricably bound to their health beliefs and behavior, as are those of many Whites. They talk a lot about "their Lord Jesus Christ" and how He came to earth for their benefit. If they just follow his Word, they feel, then a better life will be theirs. "The family of the Lord" is an important metaphor for these people and they attempt to apply it to their daily lives. It is such religious symbols, combined with their sense of family and kinship, that provide the basis for the meaning these Coberly residents give to everyday life. They provide most Blacks of Coberly with a meaning and structure.

From this tightly organized neighborhood, we move to the northeast, the area east of the courthouse. A two-lane road leading to the town of Halloday divides the rather scattered houses in this part of town in which no neighborhood exists. The Department of Family and Children Services is located less than a mile from the courthouse. A few dirt roads close to town run transverse to the main road, some leading to clusters of black houses and other clusters of white houses. These people know their proximate neighbors and often call on them for support. Most are poor, although a minority of the Whites hold semi-professional jobs. These struggling middle-class people work outside the town and most often outside the county. They are attempting to "fix up" their houses and accumulate enough wealth to buy the consumer goods they want. Others are much poorer and feel lucky to just live day by day. They are not particularly supportive of their neighbors but, like all the residents of Coberly, highly value their family and kinspeople and, at times, their religion. The family is the key support system, although some men rely on "their buddies" and the women use the activities of the church as a support resource.

As we move further east, the clusters of houses disappear and large expensive houses appear on large tracts of land. These farms and farmhouses belong to a few middle-class Whites, most of whom are of the "old families" of Coberly, and whose kinship ties are on the west side of town in the other middle-class neighborhood. The characteristics of these people are quite similar to those of their counterparts in west Coberly.

Summary

An assessment of the impact of health policy on the community level requires an understanding of the culture and structure of the people being affected by such policies. In order to explain the character of linkages, the cultural and social context in which these linkages and subsequent changes take place must be described. In this chapter, I have presented the people of Coberly, their lifestyles and county organization within the Southern regional context. The social and cultural models that have emerged in the South over the past two centuries, combined with the symbols that they use to make sense of the past and present, provide both mutable and immutable categories for their current beliefs and behavior. The people of

Coberly in many ways are a microcosm of the social models which explain their faith in the past and strong feelings of continuity with it.

There are two well-integrated neighborhoods in Coberly that have a sense of history, belonging and support. Furthermore, the people vary in their lifestyles based mainly on socioeconomic characteristics and culture. There are people who have rarely, if ever, been out of the county—and then usually only to visit kinspeople or a physician. They generally do not support radical social changes and maintain a closed worldview. Some people are more oriented to areas outside the county for parts of their lives, and they support some changes, although they remain rather conservative, with a semi-open worldview. Lastly, there are people who are regarded as "outsiders," who have an open worldview and are generally the creators of change. They develop linkages with people in the community who share some of the values, and plan to bring about changes, most of which are designed to create new jobs and to bring more wealth to the area. Many of these changes (such as the primary health care clinic) are accomplished with governmental support and thus develop a dependence on such funds, since the tax base can never support expensive programs and the people are too poor to pay fees for such services. Ironically, these new services provide resources other than kinship or religion for the people of Coberly to use as their basis for structure. The community has always been heterogeneous, but in the past, differences fitted into an overall structure and culture of the old South. In recent years, however, rural life has changed, and is beginning to look more like urban life. Much of this change is due to increased governmental services to rural areas. Coberly is no exception. It is changing, and its people are also acting and making decisions about the changes. Their decisions about health care and their linkages to the medical system vary according to their socioeconomic status and cultural models. They are not inactive players in the health arena. Their behavior is based on how they define themselves within their family, community and religion.

3

Alternative Illness
Behavior and
Decision Making

The heterogeneous nature of the population of Coberly, combined with its people's cultural background and health problems, are variables that help us make sense of its health behaviors. The term "health behavior" is used here in its broadest sense, to encompass the actions that people take when they get sick, the measures they take to stay well (including compliance with physicans' orders), their utilization patterns and their decisions about which health care system to use. Throughout this book, people are regarded as decision-makers, as purposeful actors in a hierarchy of systems. This is a crucial factor in the formulation of health policies and in providing services to people in similar contexts.

Furthermore, it is important to understand how people at the community level link to the medical system. Knowledge of these linkages can help health planners to design more effective programs, not only at the local level but at state and regional levels as well. The next three chapters explore the health behavior and beliefs of the people of Coberly.

Research Strategies
and Population Characteristics

The people of Coberly have a variety of health problems, and they respond behaviorally to these problems in patterns that vary with socio-economic status. Information on their illnesses, their health-seeking behavior and the access and utilization processes involved in their health decisions was obtained through sampling one-fourth of the households in the com-

TABLE 13
Selected Population Characteristics by Race

	White		Black	
	No. in Sample	Percent	No. in Sample	Percent
Sex (All persons interviewed)	40	54.3	34	45.7
Male	18	42.1		
Female	23	57.9	27	84.4
Age				
20–44	16	42.	12	41.9
45–64	11	23.2	11	35.5
65+	13	34.8	11	22.6
Education				
2–6	3	8.0	9	22.6
7–11	13	34.2	17	54.8
12	12	28.9	5	12.9
13+	12	28.9	2	9.7
Income				
$1,000–$5,000	4	23.5	11	40.6
$5,000–$7,500	4	10.8	5	9.4
$7,500–$10,000	3	8.1	7	15.6
$10,000–$15,000	6	16.2	5	12.6
$15,000–$20,000	5	13.5	1	3.1
$20,000+	11	29.7	0	0.
Refused	4	8.7	5	15.6

munity, interviewing key persons, and observing interactions in clinics and in key households. A total of 74 households, representing 235 people were surveyed, 55 with male household heads and 16 with female heads of household. The data collected were analyzed by comparing a number of characteristics such as age, ethnicity, sex and education. Of the 235 people on whom we collected information, 48 were between ages 0–11, 30 were ages 12–18, 54 were ages 19–34, 63 ages 35–64, and 41 were over the age of 64—a ratio that generally mirrors that in the community as a whole.

Slightly over 54 percent of the sample households are White and 45.7 percent Black (Table 13), percentages that also nearly mirror the racial makeup of the community. The educational level of those surveyed likewise reflects that of the county population, with a majority of the people, Black and White, having little or no college. Income levels reflect those of the county as well, although some respondents refused to answer the questions about income; our interpretations about income variables thus have a wider margin for error. Among those reporting income (80 percent of households), 71 percent earn below $15,000. Just over a quarter reported salaries below $5,000, 22 percent reported making between $5,000 and $10,000, and 15.5 percent said they make between $15,000 and $20,000. Only 11.5 percent reported earning above $20,000. Most of the poor and elderly (who make up a third of those interviewed) use Medicare or Medicaid as the only third-party payment source for doctors, clinics and hospitals. While 37 percent of the respondents have insurance, 18 percent pay for health services themselves. A similarly small percentage (16 percent) has hospitalization insurance only and must pay for other medical care. Twelve percent have no insurance at all.

Coberlians were interviewed about several aspects of their health and illnesses. The interview schedule was divided into five sections: (1) chronic and acute illness in the past 2 years; (2) preventive behavior; (3) mental health; (4) prenatal care and childbirth; and (5) attitudes and beliefs. The interview included questions on current health-seeking behavior and on decisions made from among the options these people feel are available to them. Hoping to find out whether different ailments were associated with different behaviors, we asked about a variety of illnesses. The interviewers (myself and four graduate students) probed interviewees about their use of alternative healing practices and in the last section, we asked questions about utilization, access, and attitudes toward doctors and "scientific" medicine.

Most people were reluctant to answer those questions related to mental health, so a great deal of care was taken to phrase these questions so that people would not be offended. I pretested this sensitive section, along with the other sections, with a concern for eliciting information that would adequately reflect the people's perspective without questioning or offending their sense of integrity and identity. Before entering the community, members of the research team, in addition to pretesting, interviewed one another and role-played a variety of responses expected from interviewees. After the interview phase began, we met weekly to discuss the interview process and any problems we encountered. In addition to structured interviewing, we visited Coberly for special events, and spent time in the clinics, the pharmacy, the center for the elderly, and the churches. We had lunch and dinner with people in the community and generally participated in community activities for eighteen months.

Illness Episodes for Chronic and Acute Illnesses

The people of Coberly experience a variety of illness episodes, both chronic and acute, that in many ways mirror the epidemiological patterns in rural areas. By far, the most frequent illness episodes—specifically hypertension, heart attacks and strokes—are related to heart problems. Most people report the usual colds, flus and children's diseases, and few have no health problems. Their decision-making process is greatly influenced by their previous illness experiences and their type of illness.

Chronic problems dominate their illness experiences. Only six households (the heads of which were all under forty years old) reported that their most serious health problems are occasional colds or the flu. Most illness episodes are an accepted part of the people's daily lives. They are anomalous occasions like other misfortunes, but are not separated out as "medical events"; instead they are treated as normal behavioral episodes. Many of the people did not understand why we were interested in such expected occurences and asked us why we would devote so much time to mundane matters.

In this chapter, the variables of socioeconomic levels, sex, and ethnicity will be used to describe and compare differences among this population's health behaviors. Correlating behavioral differences with these variables can help health care providers and policy-makers understand the different illness behavior patterns encountered in the clinical setting.

Traditional Illness Episodes Among Blacks

Seventy percent of the black sample experience problems with their heart or blood. Most described these problems with the term "high blood" and said that they were aware of this illness only because the doctor or nurse had tested them when they had been seeking care for another problem. Although their doctor had told them that hypertension is serious, they knew that the doctor and his medicines would help very little; after all, the disease has no symptoms. Very few experience problems with low blood pressure, or "low blood." Several women, however, believe that their blood has been low since miscarriages, or since their "woman's operation."

Diabetes, cognitively related to "blood problems," was reported often (31 percent of sample). Too much sugar in the blood is felt to run in the family. Diabetes is often self-diagnosed and treated with popular medicines until an acute episode occurs. At that time, the individual is taken to a physician for diagnosis. Several people said that they had probably suffered from sugar problems for years before a doctor diagnosed it. Many Blacks interviewed expect to have diabetes, especially if they have a relative with the disease. If they perceive that the symptoms occur, they will self-treat them long before it is spotted as a health problem by medical personnel.

Over 60 percent reported arthritis and rheumatism problems, the majority of which are self-diagnosed. These disorders are viewed as very similar, often lumped together in conversation. Both bring about pain in the bones and joints and are treated similarly. Many Blacks are unable to work full days or even full time because of periodic arthritic episodes. Like blood problems and diabetes, arthritis and rheumatism are accepted as a normal part of their daily lives, and adjustments to these illnesses are made as a matter of course. Similar attitudes were found with regard to some more mundane ailments, such as headaches and backaches, although very few said that these problems kept them from normal daily activities. They feel that frequent headaches (which 92 percent of respondents reported) are related to arthritis, nerves, tension, and stress, as are general aches and pains. In fact, all these illness episodes are clustered in the minds of the people of Coberly.

Likewise, stomach problems are often related to nerves, tension and stress; ulcers, on the other hand, are more frequently connected with dietary behavior than with stress. Kidney-bladder difficulties are most always related to stomach problems. Only a few self-diagnose their stomach and/or kidney-bladder problems. These problems, believed to be inherited, or to "run in the family," are often verbally described by relating stories about the problems their parents, uncles and aunts, or grandparents had suffered from such illness episodes. If the pain becomes too severe, a physician is consulted to confirm a person's diagnosis and to give him or her a shot or pill to relieve the pain.

Another kind of acute illness episode, which at times incapacitates the victim, is accidents (30 percent of respondents), mostly work-related. A majority of Blacks (both male and female) work manual jobs with a high risk of accidents. If one occurs, it often causes them to miss work for days or even weeks. Furthermore, these accidents often create chronic health problems such as arthritis.

Surgery, another illness episode that creates financial hardships, was reported only twice for black males within the past two years (for a hernia and a kidney stone) and eight times for women, all related to "female problems." A large percentage (35 percent) of the women had undergone hysterectomies, a term several of the women did not know, reporting it as a "female operation." Some reported that their doctors had told them that they should have the "female operation" for general health purposes.

Other illness episodes experienced in black households are menstrual problems, liver disorders, lung-respiratory diseases, and cancer. We had no cases of sickle cell anemia in our sample. This does not necessarily mean that these households do not suffer from this or still other health problems. They just did not report them or talk about them. Those illnesses they did discuss were overwhelmingly described with phrases or terms like "high blood," "feeling low," "nerves," "arthritis/rheumatism," "accidents," and "headaches." These terms form "core symbols" (Goode 1977) for categorizing and explaining illnesses, which will be discussed in Chapter 4. These, then, are the illnesses Blacks live with daily, those which have become a part of their lives.

These interviewees did not know the scientific terms for their illnesses and immediately translated a physician's words into their traditional categories, which have a mixed traditional/scientific etiology. As we interviewed, the same process took place. We had to translate the medical terms we used into descriptive terms that were familiar to our interviewees. In their discussions of illness, they used only a few categories to describe their symptoms. Therefore, it would appear to an outsider either, that they do not have certain illnesses, or that they are ignorant of illnesses. These encounters made it clear to me that the nature of a physician or other health care specialist's interaction with these patients is crucial, not only for correct diagnosis of an illness, but also for making accurate assessments of the incidence of disease in rural areas. These data direct health policy and health services. Communication along these linkage lines from people within the system consequently affects both health services and health behavior—a topic to be discussed in a later chapter.

Traditional Illness Episodes Among Whites

The most striking difference between the illness episodes experienced by Whites and those of Blacks involves the Whites' larger semantic domain; i.e., the wider range of terminologies used to describe illnesses. While Blacks discussed "colds," Whites frequently discussed "the flu" or "viruses" or "germs" in addition to "colds." Likewise, Whites reported problems like bronchitis, emphysema, inner ear trouble, pneumonia, appendicitis, glaucoma and cataracts. Based on these data, then, Whites appear to have a wider variety of illnesses. Although this would be a logical conclusion, observation and general participation with Blacks leads me to conclude otherwise. Such reporting reflects the differential categorization of illnesses, with Whites generally having a wider terminological system that corresponds to that of the scientific medical system.

Furthermore, there are differences between Blacks and Whites in terms of frequency of specific illnesses. The most frequently reported illness episodes for both, however, relate to heart problems. Whites suffer from hypertension or high blood pressure less often; about 20 percent reported heart trouble of some kind that caused secondary problems. One man said his "heart races," which causes his legs to swell and builds up fluid around the heart, causing the heart to hurt. Although many people related their heart problems to other physical problems, few connected them to dietary habits. Whites discussed extensively the possibility of a heart attack, usually accompanying the discussion with stories about relatives or neighbors who had suffered a heart attack. They also reported a substantially higher frequency of strokes than Blacks.

The remaining illness episodes do not cluster in the minds of Whites as do the ones discussed by Blacks. More cancer episodes were discussed among Whites than Blacks. In addition to heart problems, a majority of both groups expected that cancer would attack an immediate family member if someone else in the family had experienced the illness. Whites appeared very knowledgeable about the disease and all of them related stories of loved ones who had either died or suffered from cancer episodes. They seemed frightened by the disease and often self-diagnosed it when they detected one or two of the "warning signals" that either a physician had told them about or, more often, they had read about in magazines or heard about on television. When this occured, people would, often on the advice of a relative or friend, visit a physician. Even though they appear very concerned about cancer, relatively few people in Coberly reported cancer as a main problem.

A few people had what they called "mild cases" of diabetes. Only one, however, took medication. The Whites, like the Blacks, felt that this illness "runs in the family" and they expected that someone in their family would eventually have it. As with cancer, they self-diagnose diabetes but, unless they deem it serious, i.e., they severely suffer from what they believe are its symptoms, such as obesity, feeling faint, craving sugar and swollen legs, they do not confirm their diagnosis by visiting a physician. People who have a family member with diabetes know that they are at risk and when these general symptoms occur, they frequently just assume they have diabetes.

Another striking difference between Blacks and Whites is in the area of surgery and accidents. Over sixty-five percent of the Whites had undergone some type of surgery, compared to only two percent of Blacks. Whites often discussed their surgery, as they did cancer, in detail. They had undergone it for a variety of reasons such as abdominal problems, gall stones, hernia, cancer, hysterectomy, breast and prostate problems. Whites had experienced about the same frequency of accidents as Blacks; however, the contexts of these accidents differed significantly. Most Whites' accidents had occurred during recreational (including school) or household activities rather than work-related activities.

As with Blacks, Whites juxtaposed headaches and backaches with stress but, unlike Blacks, they also related such illness episodes to allergies and sinus problems. About ninety percent have problems with headaches/ backaches and feel that they are a "problem of life." In their extended paradigm, pain is also associated with arthritis/rheumatism, all of which is discussed as arthritis, and not as rheumatism or bursitis. Bursitis was often mentioned by Whites but was not mentioned by Blacks at all. These illnesses are chronic problems which the people cope with daily, and as such are discussed and reported frequently. These people feel that general stress and tension (very few discussed nerves), usually concerning work-related problems, are related to headaches and even allergies (although allergies and sinus problems are also inherited). Of the high percentage of Whites who reported arthritis, almost seventy percent are self-diagnosed. That is, they feel general pain and relate it to bones and joints. Other problems more infrequently experienced by Whites include kidney-bladder problems, lung/respiratory, menstrual and stomach problems. No cases of liver problems, low blood pressure or sickle cell anemia (several people did not know what this term meant) were reported by Whites.

These reported illness episodes varied by age and sex of the respondents. While illness episodes reflect age differences (i.e., arthritis and heart problems were reported only by those over 40 years old), analysis of the sex differences is more interesting and more illuminating about illness behavior and the nature of linkages men and women have to the medical system.

Traditional Female/Male Illness Episodes

The illness episodes experienced by men and women demonstrate that their perceptions of illness and illness behaviors, including recognizing and acting on symptoms, are quite different. The differences between black and white males and those between black and white females are insignificant and will not be broken out as separate categories. Sexuality, like ethnicity, proves to be a key variable in describing differences in health behaviors.

Overwhelmingly, the major illness episodes of men are problems resulting from accidents and those which concern the heart. Black and white men discussed chronic physical problems such as arthritis, often self-diagnosed, which they felt came about because of accidents, operations or "old age." Furthermore, most men said that they have headaches and stomach problems frequently. Headaches were the most frequently reported chronic problem. Many said that headaches generally came at the end of the day but since this happens so often, headaches and related arthritic pain are an accepted malady in the course of the day.

Men also expect illness episodes related to heart and blood problems. Almost eighty percent of the men reported that they suffered from hypertension. All of them are over fifty years old and discovered that they were hypertensive only because they had acute illness episodes which forced them to see a doctor. None had voluntarily had their blood pressure checked. The acute episode was frequently a stroke or heart attack (often mild), dizziness associated with headaches, or an accident of some sort. Males interviewed did not report problems with low blood pressure, diabetes, sickle cell anemia, or the liver, and only a few episodes of cancer, colon or lung/respiratory problems were recorded. The men who had had surgery, most of whom are white, reported operations for hernia, gall bladder and prostate gland. Women, on the other hand, had experienced a wider range of illnesses and generally would detail these problems more than men. Among elderly women, health problems are major topics of discussion. The most frequent episodes surround heart and blood problems, arthritis, diabetes, stomach problems, nerves and colds. The key differences between black and white women mirror the differences between the two groups in general. That is, a wider vocabulary related to illness resulting in more reported illnesses, and somewhat less concern about hypertension and diabetes, were found among white women. Black women, however, dwelled on diabetes and arthritis almost as much as heart problems.

Fewer women than men had suffered from heart attacks and strokes but about an equal number have high blood pressure. Like men, about ninety percent of women have headaches and backaches, while sixty percent said they had arthritis. And, as with the men, these problems are thought of as a part of their daily lives. Fewer women think of arthritis as a result of accidents, although, like the men, the pain usually occurs in hands and legs (knees). Headaches are related to stress and tension and, unlike men, most women have headaches throughout the day and night. A few women had gall bladder or kidney problems; fewer still had lung and respiratory problems, liver problems or cancer. Menstrual pain was discussed very little and sickle-cell anemia not at all. About forty percent of women (mostly white) had experienced surgery, mostly for breast or ovary problems. As previously stated, about twenty percent of the women had had a hysterectomy. Additional operations included colon, back and eye surgery.

Illness Response

Factors determining the responses of the people of Coberly to illness episodes include the perceived seriousness of the illness, interaction with family and/or friends to determine their collective knowledge of and experience with the illness, the perceived efficacy of the treatment, and the cost of services. In cases deemed "serious," most people either see a doctor or go to the emergency room in the nearby town. These cases include heart attacks or strokes, "serious accidents" such as car wrecks, or ones that involve unconsciousness or broken bones, and acute pain sustained over an extended period of time.

Coberlians, both black and white, respond similarly to very serious health problems, especially acute situations. When a heart attack, stroke or serious accident occurs, the household is mobilized immediately to call an ambulance or a physician or to drive the stricken individual to the hospital. Turning to the medical system is always the primary response. When there is no one in the houshould to help, friends and/or neighbors are called upon. As one respondent said, "you call the ones who care for you to help." When such an episode occurs, the relatives/friends discuss what is the best approach to take, i.e., which hospital to take the person to (the decision being based primarily upon the hospital their physician, if they have one, is using). They also discuss the cost, whether the ill person has insurance and how they will pay for the necessary services. If the ill person is female, she is consulted less on these matters than a male would be. The decision-making process is always a collective one. The choice, however, depends on the cultural and socioeconomic background of the family involved, a topic to be discussed later in this chapter and in Chapter 4.

What happens in a Coberlian household when someone suffers from an illness episode that is not perceived as serious? We found that the people of Coberly, almost without exception, rely on relatives again to take care of them. Blacks rely on their sons and daughters or other relatives, while Whites rely on their spouses more frequently. Among Blacks, family members sometimes travel from other areas, perhaps as far away as Chicago. If they do not call on their relatives, they rely on "the self"; i.e., no one is called or there is no one available to take care of the ill person and his or her household. Fifteen percent of Blacks and Whites, all below 40 years of age, fall into this category. Likewise, an equal percentage (5 percent) of both groups reported that they initially rely on doctors or the hospital (mostly the emergency room) to take care of them during an illness episode. In conversations with the people who reported doctors as a first option, it was clear that they think of this option only for serious acute episodes, not chronic illnesses or less serious illnesses like the flu.

Advice from family and friends is sought in cases of minor accidents, persistent aches and pains, or recurrent problems which they feel "doctors cannot help" or "medicines do no good" for, which are frequently treated with home remedies and over-the-counter medicines. Some opt to see a traditional healer, a person in the community who is believed to have special knowledge about illness and who usually prescribes teas, over-the-counter medicines and/or behavioral changes such as more sleep or less drinking. Many people, especially the elderly, compare doctors and medications for illnesses such as high blood pressure or arthritis and sometimes try each other's medicines. They give each other advice and, based upon their perception of the best treatment, often change their treatment from the one that has been prescribed by a doctor or nurse.

The initial social force involved in health-seeking behavior is a person's extended kin and friendship group. This social network functions to give support and to help define and validate the reality of the person experiencing illness episodes. So, describing health-seeking behavior requires an approach that is more complex than arranging responses to illness in sequences or discussing them according to degree of seriousness. Health decision-making is a discourse, a negotiation between the ill person and his/her social context, which includes all the alternatives available within the cultural framework. Over time, people's responses change as they interact with others in the community who have similar illnesses. All the people of Coberly spend a great deal of time comparing symptoms, and when an illness episode occurs that requires a new response they turn to family members first. In most cases, an older woman is chosen by both men and women. The younger people, below 30 years of age, turn to their mothers, their grandmothers or someone else in the community who knows how to treat illness. This is true even if they have to call another town or state. If this advice does not work, other avenues are sought: either friends, a pharmacist, or God. In other words, people activate different linkages in their social structure.

Through time, people learn how others cope with and overcome illness episodes. There is an informal structure of illness knowledge and response which they learn in their immediate families or, in later years, from their friends. As people age, they respond in the ways their information system has taught them, and if one response doesn't work, they will try another and another. Such pragmatism does not presume the general dichotomy of Western medicine: folk and scientific medicine. People utilize all options available in their systems of knowledge in choosing their responses; a choice based on one type of medicine does not preclude one based on the other. All responses are utilized, and some are rejected if they are not effective at a specific time. The point is, advice is sought from a variety of sources, and each suggested treatment is evaluated based on previous experience and then pursued or rejected depending on the perceived seriousness of the illness and the perceived efficacy and cost of the treatment, as we will see in the next section.

Symptom Perception and Illness Behavior

The perception and evaluation of persistent symptoms are the bases on which a decision is made to seek help from outside the popular health system; i.e., from the medical system. People in Coberly generally seek outside help when a symptom is perceived as being life-threatening or disruptive and painful, a finding similar to that of Jones, et al. (1981). Jones found also that familiarity of symptoms and perceived personal responsibility for their occurrence are significant factors in the decision to seek help. In Coberly, familiarity with symptoms is important in this decision-making process, but how the symptoms are interpreted is crucial. A symptom may be familiar and be interpreted as severe or mild. Each of these interpretations generally stimulates a response, respectively, to seek help outside the popular system or to seek advice from friends/family or from the popular system.

The symptoms experienced by the people of Coberly tell them whether a doctor's advice is necessary to solve the illness episode. Blacks reported half as many symptoms as Whites as the basis for seeing a physician. Both groups feel that a high fever and severe pain are the most common symptoms for which help must be sought. Blacks feel that not being able to go to work indicates that someone should see a doctor, while Whites rarely discussed time lost on the job. Unlike Whites, Blacks reported loss of appetite, inability to sleep, loss of a medication's effectiveness, disorientation, fainting, and choking as the key symptoms in making the decision to see a doctor or go to a clinic. Whites discussed all of these symptoms reported by Blacks, but, as previously stated, they named as many more.

Language and sequencing of multiple symptoms are other differences between Blacks and Whites in discussing their health behaviors. Blacks discussed multiple symptoms more frequently than Whites, many of which begin with "high fever." For example, "high fever and bad throat," "high fever, doesn't eat, and vomiting," or "high fever and medicine doesn't work." Upper-income Whites (over $15,000 annually) often reported fever but with more precision, such as: "symptoms last more than 24 hours with a fever about 100 degrees for more than 24 hours," "symptom severity and persistence such as fever or bleeding," "severity and length of an illness," "a complex of symptoms gets worse" or "temperature of 103 degrees for 24 hours." Blacks (all earning under $15,000) described symptoms in more behavioral terms such as "they keep lying around" or "they cannot get out of bed or move around the house." Both Blacks and Whites frequently talked about the basis for their judgement that someone is sick. The two basic criteria are "looks" and "how they act." A person who "looks" pale, weak, or different, and moves slowly, acts hysterical or disoriented, or acts like he or she is in severe pain, is considered ill.

"From whom can the people of Coberly seek help, other than a doctor?" The answers, once symptoms are perceived as serious enough to warrant obtaining help from someone, are varied and multiple, and are patterned according to ethnic background and income. A few people feel that no one can provide help other than the doctor, but most named other alternatives. A majority of Blacks believe that God or "the Lord" can help them get well and they consequently turn to "Him" through prayer. Whites named God much less frequently than Blacks; all Whites who discussed God are poor. Many reported that it is really God who is working through a doctor's hands. Next to God, the most frequently named alternatives for Blacks include "self," a healer, a person who "gives teas," "cures the thrash," or "talks fire out of burns," or home remedies. Other alternatives, less frequently named by Blacks, included minister, friends/family, nurse, pharmacist and midwife. The pharmacist was discussed rather frequently; indeed, more frequently than the nurse.

Whites also named God, but did not refer to traditional healers. A majority (85 percent) of middle- and upper-income households felt that no one can help except a doctor. Others among these groups talked about using acupuncture, a physician's assistant, naturopathy, psychiatrists and "other professional medical personnel" (including chiropractors and pharmacists) for their ailments. Some also discussed the use of herbs (such as aloe vera for constipation) and home remedies (such as sugar and kerosene for sore throat). Thus, Whites with middle-class backgrounds who do not feel that "nobody" but a doctor can help them, also use home remedies and other practitioners in a broadly defined medical system. A majority of Whites feel that they can help themselves and that family/friends, ministers and counselors can help.

Both Blacks and Whites seek help from a doctor at some time for illness episodes. Most of the people have a specific doctor they visit regularly in acute cases. The poor use the public health clinic more frequently because they cannot afford a private doctor. Furthermore, people without insurance and those who do not qualify for government help delay using the medical system, relying more on self-help. (At the time of this study, the only doctor located in the county was the one at the newly opened primary health care clinic; all others were located at least fifteen to twenty miles from Coberly.) More Blacks than Whites use the public health clinic, and Blacks tend to rely on family, friends and God for advice more frequently than Whites. On the other hand, both groups engage in self-help techniques and use the pharmacist (a white man), with Whites reporting using this alternative more often than Blacks. Whites also reported using a relative who was either a doctor or nurse, while Blacks did not.

In Coberly, illness behavior differs, then, between Blacks and Whites, although they use the same criteria for decision making. The key differences, as stated above, are rooted in the variety of options Blacks feel that they have when they are ill. Whites, while feeling they have more options to link to the established medical system, have a narrower view of their options in the non-medical domain. Furthermore, when the illness behavior is sequenced, Whites see a doctor first for both chronic and acute illnesses more often than Blacks, who seek help from other options before visiting a doctor. This is especially true for older black people who, until the past two decades, did not have doctors as an option.

Significant differences in illness behavior also exist between sexes among both Blacks and Whites. Men, when they seek help, overwhelmingly rely on doctors, while women utilize other alternatives available to them before seeing a doctor. Men are more reluctant to discuss asking family and friends for advice and when they do, it is almost always their wife or mother. Many men will endure pain for a long time rather than "go to a doctor." Several said "What can he do for me? Just make money off me." We observed several cases in which men were, in our opinion, putting themselves at a high risk for serious illness by not linking to the medical system. Women, on the other hand, discussed "turning to God," "running to the drugstore" and "asking mother," in addition to "seeing the doctor," or "going to the health clinic."

It should be pointed out, however, that the majority of both Blacks and Whites use the medical system. If a person does not initially choose a doctor, as is most often the case unless the illness is evaluated as serious, the referral chain for illness episodes includes family and/or friends, the pharmacist, God, the local healer, popular medicine (self-treatment), an emergency room physician and/or a health clinic. For example, one black woman said, "Well, first I go to mother, sometimes to the pharmacist, and then the doctor." Another said, "My husband, then God—the Good Lord and then neighbors," while another reported, "I mostly pray to God; if He doesn't help me get well and my teas do not work, I go to a doctor." Still another said, "in the past I went to the emergency room and now I go to the doctor."

The four examples below help to illustrate the variation in the ordering of available resources.

(1) Ms. Jones, a forty-three-year-old woman (black)

She feels that doctors don't help people to get well. "They administer medicine, but God heals, not doctors." During a previous illness, doctors told her to pray because they couldn't help her; God helped. Doctors don't know what is best. They are wrong sometimes. She knows what hurts and what doesn't. She follows a doctor's instructions if she deems they are good ones. If pills make her feel bad, she does not take them. Ms. Jones often opts for following the advice of a traditional healer; she also uses a variety of popular medicines.

(2) Ms. Thomas, a fifty-seven-year-old woman (black)

When she had dizzy spells, she asked her sister what she could do. The advice was to rest more, drink teas and maybe see a doctor. Ms. Thomas did and she thinks doctors helped her get well. They know what is best because they know more about medicines that make one well. But, "You don't just go see one before you've tried other remedies first."

(3) Ms. Smith, a fifty-nine-year-old woman (white)

She was told by a neighbor that she might have high blood pressure; she had it checked. Now she has it checked at the health clinic and she frequently sees her doctor. She feels that several medicines help with her condition, but you have to have confidence in the doctor you go to. Some doctors are better than others, so one should shop around to find one who can help. Other things can help, like eating better or praying more. She generally feels that the nurse at the clinic can help just as much as the doctor, unless the problem is very serious.

(4) Ms. Reed, a thirty-five-year-old woman (white)

She feels that a variety of options can help one get well, the doctor being one of them. It is basically up to the individual's mind, behavior and general outlook toward life. She uses popular medicine initially and subsequently seeks a physician's advice.

In summary, we find that Coberlians' decision-making processes involve an ordering that includes the dimensions of seriousness of illness, knowledge about it, and cost and perceived effectiveness of alternative treatments. If an illness (based on one or several symptoms) is judged as serious, more often than not both Blacks and Whites will seek out a physician, go to the public health clinic, go to the emergency room, or ask for God's help. If it is judged as non-serious, self-help via home remedies, over-the-counter drugs, the minister or traditional healers will be utilized (Figure 6). These judgements are consistent throughout the illness episodes experienced by the people of Coberly.

Preventive Health Behavior

Preventive behavior involves engaging in activities that prevent illness and disease and requires some awareness of the effects these activities have on one's health. The preventive behaviors we asked the people of Coberly about included regular checkups with physicians and dentists, tests for tuberculosis, high blood pressure checks, pap tests and other self-help behaviors they believe will help them stay healthy. The knowledge that provides the basis for their self-help and preventive behaviors comes from two sources. One is traditional medicines that they buy from the pharmacy or home remedies they learn about from family or friends. The second source of knowledge is that which comes from personnel in the medical profession, usually the public health nurse for Blacks and doctors for Whites.

Most people in Coberly utilize either some kind of medical facility in the surrounding counties or the facilities in Coberly—the public health clinic or the newly established primary health clinic—for acute problems. Many people could not remember when they had had their last health physical and most do not have physical examinations unless a specific health problem causes them to see a doctor. At the time of the study, a majority of the people had seen a doctor within the previous year. Most travel to nearby towns (between 15 and 30 miles from Coberly) to a doctor's office or to the emergency room of a hospital in a neighboring county. The poorer Blacks and Whites consult primary health clinics and the public health nurse more frequently for problems than do upper-income Whites. People with higher incomes use the public health clinic only for shots.

75

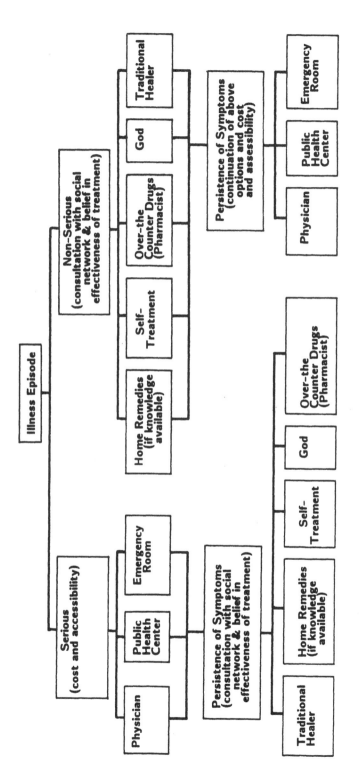

Figure 6. Health-Seeking Behavior

Women have checkups more frequently than men, and black men under the age of fifty see a doctor less often than anyone in the community. Men usually have checkups only because their jobs require it. Likewise, men usually do not see a dentist regularly, a pattern that is also shared by all low-income people of Coberly, both Black and White. The middle-income families, however, have dental checkups at least once a year and try to send their children twice a year. Most Blacks had either not seen a dentist in the past five years, or could not remember ever seeing one. Overall, 61 percent of Blacks do not have regular dental checkups and when they do or when they must see a dentist, they travel to an adjacent county, generally to the same town in which they visit a doctor.

Tuberculosis is not a serious problem in Coberly; the elderly talk about "the consumption," but only a few of the younger adults consider it a topic worth discussing. Most people do not know when they were last tested for T.B., or do not remember being tested at all. The majority of Blacks who remembered having a T.B. test said that it was done at the public health clinic. The majority of Whites thought they were tested either in a series of tests at the doctor's office, or the public health clinic, or while they were in school, or in the armed forces. A few said that "they believed" their children had been tested at school but they were not sure. In general, the people of Coberly are not very concerned with utilizing medical services to diagnose tuberculosis, with 62 percent reporting they have never had a T.B. test.

High blood pressure, on the other hand, is an object of concern and they actively seek out regular tests to determine their blood pressure. Over 80 percent of the people who have it checked do so at least once a year. Blacks are more concerned than Whites. Most remembered the exact time they had their last checkup; no one said they could not remember their last blood pressure check. Indeed, Blacks emphasized the importance of having their blood pressure checked regularly. Their doctor or "the nurse at the health clinic" told them it is important and about 60 percent go every few months, mostly to the public health clinic. We found no significant difference between men and women over 50 years of age in their participation in this preventive behavior. Men under age 50, however, are not as concerned and do not have regular checkups. Black women under 50 are more concerned and have their blood pressure checked periodically. Most of the women learned of the importance of blood pressure tests when they sought a doctor's care during pregnancy, and they have continued to have them. Many Whites did not remember when they had a blood pressure test and those who did remember said they had one when they went to the doctor for other health problems. Of course, the Whites who have a problem with high blood pressure see their doctor regularly for tests. Unlike Blacks,

80 percent of the white people of Coberly go to their doctor's office for blood pressure tests.

The same pattern holds for "getting shots." Only 20 percent of Blacks who "get shots" do so from a doctor, while the same percentage of Whites use the public health clinic. "Getting a shot" is a metaphor which to Coberlians means a quick fix for many health problems. They talk about going to the doctor or going to the clinic "to get a shot" when they feel bad. Indeed, receiving a shot and "getting pills" are the two concrete actions on the part of medical personnel that people expect from the system. However, most people are unaware of the kind of shots they get, and many are not familiar with the kinds of medicines they take, especially their side effects. Most talked in general terms about flu shots, pain shots or immunizations for their children, with a few getting allergy shots or insulin on a regular basis. Women receive more shots than men and the only difference between Blacks and Whites in terms of attitude and knowledge is the facility utilized. Coberlians are quite like the people who live in a small rural community in northern Florida, as reported by Murphree (1976). She found that these people came into a clinic and said, "I've come to get a shot," before reporting any symptoms to a nurse or physician. When they were not given shots, many believed they would not recover. Consequently, physicians would often prescribe shots when they were not necessary.

The behavior patterns of black and white women of Coberly, when and if they have pap tests, reflects the split between doctor's offices and the public health clinic. No white women reported going to the clinic for a pap test, while about 40 percent of the black women utilize the "health department" or "medical center" (public health clinic), with the rest having their tests in a doctor's office. Fifty-three of all the women interviewed have had a pap test, with 85 percent of Whites having one every year and less than half of Blacks having had one within the past year. The remaining black women have never had a pap test or had one only when their children were born. They do not regularly have such tests and expressed little or no concern with having them. White women, on the other hand, especially those from higher income brackets, demonstrated a concern about having the test on a regular basis. All of them have a test every year. The case is different for poor white women, however. Many could not remember their last tests or said that they had never had a pap test. They did not demonstrate any knowledge about the purpose of such a test or its effect on their health.

The preventive health patterns, as defined by the medical model in Coberly, demonstrate that distinctive behaviors exist between income groups, with poor Whites and Blacks sharing similar patterns, while middle- and upper-income Whites exhibit patterns that conform to the teachings of modern medicine. The upper-income people of Coberly utilize doctors and dentists for their health problems on a regular basis, and they visit their doctors for regular checkups and for preventive measures such as pap tests and high blood pressure tests. When they use the health clinic, it is primarily for shots. On the other hand, the lower-income people of Coberly seldom have checkups with doctors and use the public health clinic more often for their health problems. They see the dentist less frequently than those in the upper income level. Blacks (especially black women) are concerned with high blood pressure more than Whites and demonstrate their concern by having frequent blood pressure tests. White women, on the other hand, are concerned more with cancer and have pap and breast tests on a regular basis. The group most concerned about high blood pressure is women 50 years old or older, and the least concerned groups for high blood pressure are black and white men, and for cancer, black men. All groups have little concern for tuberculosis.

Utilization of and Access to Medical Facilities

The community of Coberly has continuously had the services of a doctor since the 1930s, with the exception of the years 1972-1981. Since most of the people have lived their entire lives in Cober County, (some have never even been to Magnolia), most of the people are accustomed to having a doctor in town, although the poor, and most Blacks did not have access to him until the 1960s. As we saw in the last section, however, most people at the present time will, if they choose to, use a physician. There are, however, some significant differences in this regard between the sexes of both ethnic groups. A higher percentage of females than males have a regular doctor (63 percent for Whites and 71 percent for Blacks as compared to 23.7 for Whites and 18.2 for Blacks). Most Blacks have only had a regular doctor during the past ten or fifteen years. "In the old days" (1930s, 40s, and 50s), they would either "take care of themselves with the help of special people in the neighborhood and God" or "we just used the health department." Another, very recent option for them is the new primary health care clinic that opened in 1983. At the time of the study, it was in the process of beginning services to the people of Cober County. This process will be examined in a later chapter.

Whites are split half and half on whether they would use this new clinic only for emergencies. When asked to name the situations, other than emergencies, for which they might use the clinic, they included problems with their children, blood pressure checks, getting blood and if the family doctor is out of town. A few said that they would consider using the clinic only if a white doctor worked there. About fifty percent said they wouldn't use the clinic at all because they trusted and preferred their family doctor, while the other fifty percent said they would use it only under some of the circumstances noted above. A few respondents were unaware that the clinic existed, and some felt that the clinic was not needed.

Conversely, about sixty-five percent of Blacks said they used or would use the primary health clinic. Their reasons are these: (1) it is closer, (2) it is more convenient and they feel that it is cheaper than going to a private doctor, and (3) they like the doctor. The Blacks who said they would not use it, like the Whites, like and trust their own doctor. About twenty percent are unsure about using the clinic, mainly because they are afraid the doctor will not stay in the town and then they would have to change doctors again. Furthermore, many Blacks and some Whites stated that they liked the services provided by the nurse practitioner and felt that she could help them with many of those health problems for which a doctor is not needed. Both Blacks and Whites expressed their approval of the convenience of the clinic. No one who made over $10,000 reported that they used the clinic or would use it (except in extreme emergencies), while over 90 percent of those who use it or would use it have incomes of under $7,000 annually.

Although the people of Coberly talked about the convenience of the clinic and its nearness to their homes, very few feel that transportation is a problem in seeking a doctor outside the county. Only one white family reported a problem with transportation, while 3 black households said that finding someone to take them is sometimes a problem. All of these households are poor and said that the gas money ($8-$10) or the bus fare cost too much. The remaining people depend on relatives and/or friends to take them to their doctor.

Although Coberlians use the town's medical facilities frequently, they feel that there are still numerous health needs in the community. By far the most frequently reported need is a doctor; not just any doctor but a "good doctor," "a stable doctor," or "one who lives in the town." Several people discussed the problems they have in communicating with doctors and some are afraid to visit one. They want one whom they trust and have confidence in and who will stay in the town. The second most frequently reported need is an ambulance service in case of emergencies. Presently, it takes about 45 minutes for the paramedics to drive to Coberly and then back to the hospital in Magnolia. So, a permanent doctor for emergencies and emergency services in the town are perceived as the two most important medical needs in Coberly, whose people feel that improved access to hospitals and a doctor would lessen the risk of serious injury or death in emergency cases.

The third most frequently reported need relates to food, nutrition, and money to purchase the "right kind of food." Both poor Whites and Blacks feel that they are blocked from "access to food." By this, they mean more nutritious food, places to purchase it and the money with which to buy it. This was a surprising finding which indicates to me that many people are aware of the relationship between diet and health. Wherever this knowledge is obtained (public health nurse, agricultural extension agent and/or media), many people in Coberly feel that if they had access to better food, they would be healthier. Some people with upper-level incomes feel that the lack of grocery stores is a major health problem in Coberly.

Generally, Whites see a wider variety of health needs in the community than Blacks. About ten percent of Blacks and Whites reported that they do not know what the health problems are in the area. Needs discussed by Blacks, in addition to the ones noted above, are a dentist, a hospital, recreational facilities, alcohol, drug abuse programs, and more belief in God. Whites said that there is a need for a dentist, someone to deal with problems with alcoholism and drugs, and someone to provide more activities for young people. They also feel there is a need for birth control information, an improved water system, programs for senior citizens, paramedics, and a psychologist. Again, the answers of the Whites are indicative of broader knowledge about health care alternatives within the scientific medical system.

Comparative Linkages and Alternatives

In Coberly, the perceived available alternative responses to illness are based on the following: (1) people having to cope with more chronic illness episodes as they become older; (2) people having to use traditional modalities because they are poor and have not had access to "scientific" medicine; and (3) people expanding their health repertoires to include newer modalities such as chiropractors and acupuncturists because they can afford them. These responses depend on people's possible linkages to the social structure and their interpretations of these possible linkages. This is a logical finding, but is one that is not accurately reported in medical literature. Earlier studies reporting social and ethnic differences in responses to illness have not addressed the complexity of this concept, nor framed their findings within the broader systems to which people link. For example, Koos found in 1954 that upper-class people in Regionville, USA reported more illnesses than lower-class people and that they were more likely to seek medical treatment. Lower-class persons, however, had more symptoms of sickness. Likewise, Sanders (1954), in the same year found differences in the response to illness and utilization of medical facilities among "Anglos" and Spanish-speaking people in the American Southwest. Studies by Zborowski (1952, 1969) and Apple (1960) confirm these earlier studies and suggest that factors such as interference with usual activities, degree of severity, and ethnic, religious and educational background of the individual's group influence illness behavior.

Suchman (1965) delineated a number of important factors related to the social organization of the group to which an individual belongs and his/her illness responses. They include: (1) extent of knowledge of illness, (2) degree of delay in seeking treatment, and (3) use of home remedies or patent medicines. Based on his research and the general concept of the sick role (Sigerist 1960 and Parsons 1951), he formulated stages of illness experience. The stages are (1) symptom experience, (2) assumption of the sick role, (3) medical care contact, (4) dependent-patient role, and (5) recovery and rehabilitation. His model, based on the assumption of the Western medical system, attempts to describe the sequence of behavior as an individual moves from perceiving symptoms, evaluating and responding to them through the sick role (in which the individual confers with family/friends and perhaps tries self-treatment and home remedies—the lay care system) to the professional care system where the individual becomes a patient, renounces the sick role and his/her dependency and recovers or is rehabilitated.

A classic paper by Mechanic (1961) sets forth the concept of illness behavior as a further attempt to understand the varied responses to illness. He defines this term as "the ways in which given symptoms may be differentially perceived, evaluated and acted (or not acted) upon by different kinds of groups" (1961:189). He feels that "whether a person does or does not assume the sick role when ill is dependent on a variety of group and personal factors. The person's age, sex, position in his group as well as the importance of his role for the group must be considered" (1961:190). Furthermore, the person's learned behavior or what Fabrega (1973) calls the "cultural definition of symptoms," and the individual's ability to respond (access, cost) are additional factors that influence illness behavior.

Mechanic suggests four important decisions for analyzing illness behavior, the first two referring to the problem of "illness recognition" (the frequency with which the illness occurs and the familiarity of the symptoms) and the latter two "illness danger" (the predictability of the outcome and the amount of threat and loss that result from the illness). These dimensions are more helpful than Suchman's stages in explaining the illness responses and health-seeking behaviors of the people of Coberly. As Mechanic found, we see that people respond differently to those illnesses they perceive as "routine" than to the ones they perceive as "non-routine." These routine ones are mostly chronic diseases, the ones they are "use to living with" and which are generally less frequently reported.

Evaluating and acting upon symptoms is a subjective experience on the part of the individual that depends on all the factors mentioned above. To medical personnel, symptoms are understood in terms of how the human organism functions or malfunctions, but this knowledge is extremely complex and very few people understand it. This leads to the question: How do the people of Coberly understand, evaluate and act upon their symptoms?

The answer: They experiment. But they experiment with options broader than those the medical model has to offer. Experimentation is based on their experiences or those of their family and friends who have had similar illnesses. Where does their information come from? This is a more difficult question to answer because the answer varies according to age, sex, ethnicity, income and experience. An individual's knowledge of illness, description of illnesses and type of illness episodes depends on that individual's general education, contact with the professional medical system, exposure to the media (especially relevant to self-diagnosis) and beliefs and values.

The model presented by Suchman is too static to perfectly account for the illness behaviors encountered in Coberly. An individual often experiences more than one of Suchman's stages at one time, especially as he/she moves through the life-cycle. Furthermore, many people of Coberly do not pass through all these stages with one illness. Indeed, Suchman seems to be presenting us with a disease model rather than an illness model and fails to account for the "stream of illness behavior" of the elderly and of most of the chronically ill in Coberly.

In reporting symptoms, the people of Coberly report illness episodes and illness responses based on their own cultural and social context. Their experiences are shaped by their age, sex, ethnic background and income; all these factors help define and shape the cultural experience, meaning and interpretation of symptoms, the treatment selected and the degree of compliance with the chosen treatment. When experiencing an illness, an individual uses lay consultation with family/friends and follows a referral chain that varies according to the meaning of the specific symptom experience. Thus, in the sociocultural construction of symptom and illness reality, individuals in Coberly have different categories and labels for illness. These categories, or illness models are important for choosing options; they provide a symbolic collectivity between individuals, their group affiliation and the larger (medical) institutions which provide explanations and make sense out of the illness. In other words, Coberlians link to the medical system differently. Their specific illness beliefs and explanatory models will be discussed in Chapter 5.

My findings are roughly similar to those reported by Chrisman (1976), who follows the writing of Freidson (1970) in reporting American patterns of help-seeking behavior. Chrisman distinguishes between the scientific, lay and traditional health systems, and in his analysis emphasizes the lay referral system. Freidson (1970) divides the lay system into a cohesive one (more characteristic of the lower class) and an extended and closed one (more characteristic of higher social classes). The former is termed "parochial" (closed system of contacts) while the latter is called "cosmopolitan" (a wider variety of contacts). Chrisman's data is based on interviews with 14 new patients in a family practice clinic near a large university. His findings indicate that all but one of the persons were "cosmopolitan" and only one sought care immediately upon the appearance of symptoms, although all valued consulting a doctor when they had health problems. The symptoms were first discussed with family/friends for the purpose of getting advice. A second kind of information-gathering experience was interaction with the doctor. Chrisman concluded that "much of their behavior in the lay health system is directly related to the scientific health practitioners" (1976:214). The doctor is a mediating factor between the lay system of knowledge and the medical system of knowledge.

In Coberly, middle- and upper-income Whites can be characterized as "cosmopolitan," with more linkages to the established health care system, while Blacks (all poor) and poor Whites can be characterized as somewhere between "parochial" and "cosmopolitan," with fewer linkages to the established health care system. Most Whites, however, draw upon the broad "scientific" health system for their knowledge. They are aware of more categories of illness and symptoms than Blacks, but they have fewer options for illness responses and health maintenance. On the other hand, Blacks respond just as quickly as Whites in seeking a doctor for health problems and they value having a doctor. Many said that "it is not like the old days when we could not see a doctor." This option is a consistent part of their repertoire, however, only since the passage of Medicare legislation. As a consequence, the old options of traditional medicine's well-defined lay referral system are still included in their knowledge system, and, when combined with their increasing knowledge of the medical system, make Blacks' health system broader than that of Whites. In the past, Blacks depended more on people from their own support group who specialized in healing specific illnesses. My findings indicate that in some ways poor Blacks and Whites are similar in their perceptions of options (or lack of options) in their illness behavior and preferred treatment, while they are dissimilar in their overall knowledge of the scientific system and in their evaluation of symptoms.

The meaning of experienced symptoms is the guide in deciding whether to seek help from medical personnel or to use options outside the medical system. This assignment of meaning involves a disparate set of symbols (symptoms) during a given illness episode, which are linked together, mesh into an association, and then lead to a specific action (decision). The association of symbols which triggers concrete decisions is based on the knowledge and experience that the people of Coberly share. But, as we have seen, not all of the people share the same symbolic associations, depending on their level of social interaction in the social structure. As a result of their differential relationships (linkages) to their social and cultural environment, Coberlians make different associations of symptoms and consequently different decisions to seek help.

Symbolic associations are based on the dynamic system of beliefs held by the people of Coberly: dynamic because, as additional information is added to the knowledge system, bits and pieces are integrated into their explanatory models. Berkanovic, et al. (1981) found in a study of symptom experience, that network influences and personal beliefs specific to symptoms accounted for almost all of the responses to symptoms. They expressed surprise at these findings and indeed found them "disturbing." They state that "the three major predictor variables are all symptom-related [not need]. Further, the failure of either the demographic or structure of care variables to account for much variance in the decision to seek care is troublesome" (1981:707). These authors feel that their findings lend strong support to the Health Belief Model. This is disturbing to them because the findings "offer no insights into how either social structure or prior experience influences decision" and "neither [do these findings] advance our under-standing of any regularity that might underlie such behavior . . . " (1981:709). To an anthropologist, these findings are not surprising, nor are they unilluminating. Social and cultural patterns are always changing and behavior cannot be accounted for by static models of the social structure which are not explanatory, only descriptive. We have to look beyond such models to the explanatory models of the variables used to decide on specific action in seeking health care. Only then can we predict the choices people make within their social and cultural environment. This environment includes both the scientific and popular approaches to health and, to use the words of Goode:

> provides a language passed on from generation to generation, in which people voice their experience of disease. And it provides a set of ideas, cognitive models, expectations, and norms that guide the responses to disease by a patient and by those persons in the patient's home, family and neighborhood who care for him. In this way, the popular and the scientific systems of medicine socially and meaningfully construct the experience of disease and the case of the ill (Goode 1977:30).

4

Family, Community,
and Mental Health

The illness behavior patterns of the people of Coberly demonstrate that they are active decision-makers in linking to the medical system. They also demonstrate the importance of family and community in this town. The family and the household are the major units of interaction in Coberlians' lives and most families are extended into the community and the region, as are most other resources and services. Being a rural dweller means traveling within the boundaries of a specific region for shopping, health needs and jobs. The boundaries, both geographical and behavioral, are defined by the ethos of the community.

Community behavior, both public and private, differs significantly between Blacks and Whites in Coberly, where the racial boundaries that have permeated the rural South for a century can still be observed. Some rules have undergone modification within the past decade or so; the school, for example, is integrated. Churches and voluntary organizations however, remain segregated. Both Blacks and Whites can eat at the local restaurant and other public places, but leadership positions for Blacks remain mostly within the domain of the church, not the government. The health system, the banks, and the newspapers are dominated by Whites. One rarely observes members of the two groups interacting except at times when business (private or public) demands it, when specific alliances are needed to pass county or city ordinances, or when other political activities between the two groups take place. These activities reflect traditional forms of linkage in the South, which were established mainly through economic and political ties.

Each group has its own status system and, although Blacks' and Whites' cultural frameworks overlap, as in the case of health behavior and beliefs, there are many differences in the culture and structure of their places in the community. The stratification system in rural areas in general is highly complex. It is composed of extensive interconnecting relationships, formal and informal lines of communication and well-established rules of appropriate behavior. Whites base their status on family, wealth, occupation and education, while Blacks base their status more on family, since all are poor and relatively undereducated in Coberly. The kinship group to which a person belongs is important to both groups; one's family name can go a long way (toward respect and getting credit). Among Blacks, however, respect is also achieved through exhibiting the respectable behavioral patterns dictated by the community. These patterns include working hard, participating in voluntary organizations (most of which are organized through the church), believing in God and trying to live a Christian life. The latter includes not drinking in public or getting into fights, and helping out people in need. Respect is often associated with a sense of cooperation, especially within the household unit. People who are generally disrespected are those who break God's laws by drinking too much, taking drugs, remaining unemployed without attempting to find a job, having babies without a spouse and, of course, failing to participate in cooperative activities within the household or family. Older Blacks talked a great deal, however, about the fact that the sense of obligations that existed in the past no longer exists today. They lamented that the family is falling apart and "you just can't depend on people like you used to."

Whites base their respect for others more on occupation, income and education, as well as family. Most of the land is owned by white families and is passed from generation to generation. One of the most prominent white families owns a very large farm with a plantation-like house overlooking a large lake. Inside the house, one finds among the furnishings books that depict the "Old South." A member of this family has been a state senator for years. White newcomers in the community who can be classified as middle class are judged according to their jobs and income, although few are ever accepted within "the community." Only middle and upper income Whites and a few Blacks have a worldview that goes beyond the region. Indeed, we interviewed several people who had never been to the major urban area sixty miles away. As a result, they are unaware of how to activiate linkages to systems outside their structural worldview if, indeed, they are knowledgeable of them.

The family is the crucial social institution in the lives of all people in Coberly. All cultural and social forms are understood through this unit. In Hopewell, a community less than forty miles away from Coberly, Greenhouse (1986) found that the family is the link between nature and culture. She states, "It is the link between the world of men and God's heaven. It is the standard by which they measure all legitimate authority, all an individual's maturity. The family is by definition authentic: While other groups of people might feel 'like' family, 'family' itself is not qualifiable. Families . . . might be good or bad, but their goodness and badness flows from the fact that a family is literally essential" (1986:48). In the domain of health, the illness behaviors of Coberlians reflect the importance of family in responding to illness episodes. It is the only "natural unit" since it is preordained by God. Indeed, Greenhouse feels that society itself is the family "writ large." In her analysis of family religion conflict resolution, she states further that:

> The family is the smallest social unit, a unit which admits no subdivisions nor any outside intervention. Thus, families have a political autonomy in the local conception; however, balancing that autonomy is the utilitarian view that families yield some of their autonomy to the community and, through communities, to the state for their own protection. It should be noted that this is a very limited source of concession to the community, and that the subject of what local governments and other governments can demand of private citizens is a frequent one. The family is the traditional, if somewhat idiomatic, bulwark of the individual against the state: the local view is that no one, official or not, has the right to tell a man how to run his family. The family is the sanctuary of the individual against the community. . . . Families remain inviolable with this system not so much because they are understood to have divergent interests (which is the logic of democracy) but because they have a natural right to be treated as discrete decision-making units. Families form micropolitical systems, and much of the local ambivalence about social or civic authority is expressed in terms of preserving the natural and rightful autonomy of the family (1986:50).

The involvement of the family in making decisions concerning illness behavior was clearly illustrated in Chapter 3. In this chapter, health behavior in the area of health promotion (health-seeking behavior) and mental disorders will be examined within the context of community and family to further demonstrate the importance of recognizing the culture and structure of a community in planning and implementing health services.

Family and Community Linkages Throughout Life: Health-Seeking Behavior

In order to demonstrate how the people of Coberly link to one another and to the health system, the typical life cycle will be described with reference to the differences and similarities between Blacks and Whites. For both populations, the key domestic structures are the family and household, which function as the basic economic units. Heads of household are usually men, among both Blacks and Whites, although in many cases among the Blacks, a woman plays this role if she has a steady job. In Coberly many households are made up of only an elderly couple, a single elderly person, or three-generational families, often with an elderly woman, her son or daughter, his/her spouse and their children. The latter is a long-time pattern among Blacks and the exact composition of a household depends on its inhabitants' phase in the life cycle.

Women's behavior during pregnancy and childbirth reflects patterns that vary according to their age, socioeconomic level and ethnic group membership. As was true of other aspects of health behavior, the women of Coberly respond surprisingly differently to needs associated with maternal care and childbirth. As discussed in Chapter 2, the infant mortality rate among the Black population is high, much higher than the rate for Whites. A major reason for the discrepancy is a lack of prenatal and postnatal care and the dietary patterns of the mothers and children. There are questions of access to care and quality of care: linkage problems for expecting mothers and children.

Pregnancy and Infant Care

Knowing one is pregnant depends on the interpretation of changed bodiliy functions, signalled by certain events such as missing a menstrual period or experiencing nausea. Indeed, these are the two changes most frequently discussed by both black and white women. Over 80 percent of Blacks focused on "missed periods" and about half of the Whites reported "skipping a month," combined with nausea, morning sickness, and/or sore breasts. Once they suspect a pregnancy, the women of Coberly mostly ask their mothers, grandmothers and aunts for advice. Ninety percent of the black women said that the only person they ask for health-seeking advice is their mother or grandmother, with the remaining 10 percent looking beyond the family to the nurse at the public health clinic or a midwife. A majority of older black women preferred a midwife and "would never think of using a hospital." Only five percent of Blacks (all under 40 years old) use a doctor regularly during pregnancy. On the other hand, over 60 percent of the Whites said they saw a doctor regularly during pregnancy. Like Blacks, however, all ask their mothers or neighbors/friends for advice about pregnancy behavior. Although only 20 percent of black and white women change their diet during pregnancy, about 50 percent take "medicines." More Whites than Blacks take vitamins, iron and calcium when pregnant. Blacks take castor oil and epsom salts every week or so; most feel that taking vitamins would be "a good thing," but rarely do so. More than 50 percent of the Blacks said that they do not take any medicines, a majority saying they could not afford to buy them. Our observations in their households revealed that most do not have any vitamin or mineral supplements in their households, nor do they change their diets. While none of the poor (Black or White) perceive a relationship between their diets and the health of their babies, Whites with higher incomes discussed the merits of taking vitamins and minerals, for their own health as well as the health of their babies. All of the women who supplement their diets said that their doctor recommended it. "If he hadn't told me, I would never have done it."

Most white women went to see the doctor within the first three months of pregnancy; fewer than five percent reported not seeing a doctor or nurse while pregnant. On the other hand, 15 percent of the Blacks said that they never consulted a doctor or nurse during pregnancy. Blacks used the public health clinic more than doctors and generally went in their third or fourth month of pregnancy. Only persons with higher incomes made regular visits to medical personnel. Furthermore, all but one of the white women had their babies in a hospital while only 38 percent of black women had their babies in hospitals (all were under 50 years of age). Of the remaining 62 percent, 45 percent used a midwife at home, and 18 percent used a doctor at home or went to a clinic for delivery. Blacks simply cannot afford prenatal care and hospital deliveries. The system will not accept them unless they can pay. Many are turned away; consequently, we find high rates of infant mortality among Blacks.

After their babies are born, the white women of Coberly uniformly seek care from a doctor. During the interviews, none mentioned the health nurse and only two said that they did not take their babies to anyone. Black women named the public health nurse more often, with 40 percent also seeing a doctor at least one time. A few said they used a midwife and/or their mothers for consultation after their babies were born. In fact, most women depend almost entirely on their mothers and/or other relatives for advice about and care of their babies.

The time when they first used a doctor or nurse appears not to vary with ethnic group. Most women who reported having taken their babies to medical personnel did so within the first two months. A small percentage said that their children were of school age before they saw a doctor and/or nurse (all these women were over 50 years old), and a few took their children only when they were ill; they did not see any reason to go otherwise. During the first few years of their children's lives, white women utilize doctors on a regular basis for checkups, shots, etc., while black women overwhelmingly use the public health clinic for such preventive care. For 10 percent of the sample, their children did not receive medical care until they started school, after the initial visit when the baby was born.

Having a baby in Coberly is a major happening. It means adding to the family, providing new members of this "natural group." Special social occasions (baby showers and parties) ritualistically inform the community that it will be expanding. Having a baby also means that the expectant mother will link to a medical system, if only briefly, for advice and attention. The key person(s) on which a prospective mother relies is usually someone from the first ascending generation. Whites link more frequently than Blacks to the medical system and, more often than not, the two groups link to different parts of it—Blacks to public health clinics and Whites to a physician. Utilization of doctors for prenatal and postnatal care is clearly a function of income. Blacks and the poor use the public health clinics, while middle-class Whites use doctors and exhibit more concern about and awareness of the consequences of such care. In recent years, however, more Blacks have begun using the medical system, not so much for counseling during pregnancy or for postnatal care, but for delivery in hospitals or for family planning.

Child and Adolescent Health

Within the family and household, the mother or sometimes an older sibling is responsible for the care of children when they are sick. If the illness is not serious, mothers send their children to school anyway; if it is deemed serious, they either stay home (if they work) or call a relative or friend to stay with the sick child. A few require an older sibling (if one exists) to stay home from school to take care of the sick child. If the illness is more serious, based on certain symptoms such as high fever, they opt to take the child to a doctor or the public health clinic. Otherwise, the child is given various home remedies or over-the-counter medicines, as described in the next chapter. Since the unemployment rate in Coberly is high, there is generally little problem in many families about who will take care of a sick child. Although we did not correlate the frequency of illness for children of unemployed parents, Margolis and Farran (1981) found these children at greater risk for illnesses, infections, diseases and illnesses of longer duration. Very little or no attention is paid to the diet of children and teenagers. They share the food with the entire household and sneak a great deal outside the household setting. There are only two fast-food restaurants in Coberly; they are frequented by teenagers after school hours. There, as at home, teenagers consume what is considered "junk food," without much attention paid to the relationship between diet and health. Since their parent or parents for the most part are not aware of this relationship (with the exception, of course, of not eating too many sweets), young people are not socialized into healthy dietary habits. Some information is provided in a few of the courses in the high school, but it appears that their environment as a whole fosters the traditional dietary patterns of a Southern community. As a consequence, they do not have much incentive to change their eating patterns.

Most children of Coberly begin participating in the medical system upon going to school. Because of the requirements of the educational system, they then receive immunizations and checkups, primarily from the Cober County Public Health Department. The public health nurse visits the high school once or twice a year to discuss family planning. She mainly talks about the moral aspects and religious consequences of having sexual relations before marriage. Very little time is spent on anatomy and virtually nothing is said about techniques of birth control.

Adolescents receive very little information about sexual practices, either at school or in the home. Teenage pregnancy is a problem in Cober County, but because of the traditional values and attitudes of the people, a strong sex education program has not been implemented in the school. Furthermore, sexuality is rarely discussed in households with teenage children, who are thus left with the "trial and error" method by which to learn about the consequences of sexual activities.

Specific data were not available on sexual and physical abuse of children in Coberly. From state-level data, however, we find that between 1975 and 1979, 739 confirmed cases of sexual abuse and 3486 confirmed cases of non-sexual physical abuse were reported. Thus, sexual abuse accounted for 17 percent of all confirmed child abuse reports. Based on the demographic and socioeconomic characteristics of the perpetrators and victims, Janson reports that "the populations assessed as being at increased risk for sexual abuse were poor rural white children and black children living in households where the mother was the only head of household" (Janson, et al. 1982:3347). Indeed, "rural whites living below the poverty level had 4.1 times the number of confirmed physical abuse reports expected" (1982:3347). While we did not observe any episodes of physical and sexual abuse in families, we did ask questions about the people's knowledge of such behavior, reported in the section on mental health. This data indicated that the children of Coberly are at risk for being victims of abuse.

Most young people leave the county in their late teens seeking jobs, or marry an outsider and move to another town. A local joke indicating awareness of this youth drain holds that the major export in Cober County is the young people. Some will return intermittently to live, while most come home only for important ritual occasions. They sometimes send money to their parents and keep in contact with members of their families who remain in Coberly. Young and middle-aged adults comprise the smallest age group in Coberly. They have a variety of jobs, depending on their status in the community, and continue to live their daily lives often under stress, both economically and socially. As discussed in Chapter 3, they take actions and make decisions about their health, and some adults see a relationship between their work and their health.

Work, Lifestyle, and Health

Very few people in Coberly have jobs that would be categorized as professional. Conforming to the patterns of other small Southern communities, upper income Whites have jobs typically called "white collar," or professional, while lower income Whites and most Blacks hold "blue collar" or manual labor jobs. A large percentage of our sample (18 percent) is retired, and 18 percent of the Blacks are unemployed, while fewer than five percent of Whites are unemployed. Whites have "white collar" jobs— sales manager for a machinery company, purchasing agent in a machine shop or assistant manager at a K-Mart—or hold professional positions as teachers, lawyers, accountants or paramedics. About 40 percent hold jobs in mills or nearby plants or are self-employed in the craft or repair areas. About 20 percent of white women are housewives, while the others hold jobs as, for example, teachers, secretaries, nurse mill workers, or seamstresses. On the other hand, about 40 percent of the black women who are employed work in a factory or mill, while the remainder work as maids, cooks or teachers (the latter being the only professional job among Blacks). Other work includes "a little farming," working as a seamstress or mechanic, and "odd jobs" relating to yardwork and cleaning house.

Most of the women of Coberly are employed, or have been employed at one time in their lives. "Work" has a different meaning to men and women and to the different income groups. It is expected that men should have jobs and provide for their families. Black men, however, have difficulty finding jobs, and consequently many are unemployed. Black women can find jobs more easily, and thus are often the main source of income in the household. While many Blacks are on welfare, they did not readily discuss this source of income. Some Whites also receive welfare and they too, were reluctant to discuss it with us. The upper income white women who have jobs are generally professionals or work "part-time." In middle and lower income white households, both spouses hold jobs "to make ends meet."

The relationship between work activities and health is differentially perceived by the people of Coberly. Earlier, I stated that men develop chronic problems such as arthritis due to work-related accidents. Many are aware that their jobs affect their health. In one sample, 40 percent of men and women replied that they felt their work situation was detrimental to staying healthy. However, when responses were broken down into income groups, we found very little perceived relationship between health and work among lower income people. Over 90 percent said work does not influence their health, while over 50 percent of upper income people feel it does. Work seems to be an isolated behavioral category for the lower income group. They never discussed how such activities affected other parts of their lives except for references to "being tired" or "not making enough money." Upper income respondents discussed the stressfulness of their jobs and the ways stress affects their relationships and emotions. They consequently try to reduce stress in various ways; some take drugs, others have a drink or two, still others exercise or try to relax by watching television. The middle and lower income people often reported "nerve problems," but rarely related them to work.

Their response to problems with job-related stress and "nerves" varies from doing nothing (the majority of people) to taking narcotics. Whites take Valium and Librium, while Blacks just call their treatment "nerve pills." Other health management behavior of Whites includes taking aspirin, taking Doan's Pills, getting away from the problem for a while, watching television, drinking and exercising. Blacks take aspirin and "Goody's," drink, make teas, and pray. Overall, stress management is not as much thought about as acted upon among the people of Coberly. They do, however, think about preventive care and make decisions according to their ideas about what makes one healthy.

Fewer than half of the men and women overall feel that their work affects their health, and of these most think that any negative effects stem from such factors as stress/nerves, pollution (such as chemicals in plants and factories) and accidents. Less frequently discussed negative effects are tiredness, boredom, exposure to weather conditions, and eye strain. The only positive impact of their jobs on health, they feel, is the exercise they get on the job. As stated before, men relate accidents and stress as negative impacts and exercise as a positive one, while women emphasize the effects of pollution and stress. Blacks more than Whites feel that their jobs affect their health in concrete ways, and consequently when interviewed named a wider variety of impacts than Whites. In addition to stress, Blacks associate boredom, working conditions, weather conditions, colds and tiredness as job-related health factors. Very few Whites discussed these factors.

Most people of Coberly experience some kind of stress and manage it through several culturally acceptable behaviors. Over half of the people are aware of what they call "nerve problems." They believe that their stress or case of "nerves" is generally caused by work-related problems, not family problems. Some, mostly the poor, feel that their inability to purchase the items (including food) they want and/or need causes stress. "Always thinking about how we will buy the right kind of food or pay our heating bills," is a common concern among the poor. Their perception of "stress" or "nerves" is not cognitively related to "mental health" in the sense of medical categories; there is very little connection between alcoholism, drug problems or mental illness and stress in our interviews with all groups in Coberly.

Managing one's health care is an idea that many of the people of Coberly think about and act upon in a variety of ways. Although most utilize medical resources for curative and selected preventive purposes, as discussed in Chapter 3, other behaviors which are thought to ensure health involve the family and community but rarely link to the medical system. In addition to using home remedies and over-the-counter medicines and consulting persons perceived as knowledgeable about health problems, many Coberlians engage in other behaviors they believe will help them stay healthy. Although 20 percent of Blacks and Whites believe that nothing beyond medical help and home remedies will aid in maintaining one's health, the remaining 80 percent engage in a variety of behaviors and activities, which they believe directly relate to their health status. While some of the "medicines" they use technically fall into the category of home remedies, they were discussed within the context of preventive behaviors.

Men usually talked about exercise as an extension of medical help while women more frequently talked about taking vitamins. The forms of exercise men take part in are walking, working and playing sports. Another health-related activity Coberlians feel to be important is choosing the kinds of foods they eat. For example, a White woman said she "tries not to eat sweets and starches but eat more natural foods, grown in the garden, especially vegetables." Other activities the people of Coberly feel affect health include getting plenty of sleep, taking tonics and laxatives, drinking yellow root and rabbit tea, dipping snuff and praying.

Diet and Nutrition

Shopping for food is almost entirely the domain of women in Coberly. Women who do not have jobs generally go to town once a day to purchase the necessary food items for supper (the night meal). Going to the store means more than just buying food; it is also often the only time some women get out of the house or see other people during the day. Of course, the shopkeepers know their customers well; many have known one another for years. Often, a store will give specific persons credit. Such stores generally have higher prices, and thus many low income families stay in debt for their food.

Exchanges of food were rarely observed, or reported by the people of Coberly; such exchanges take place mostly between children and their elderly parents. During family crises, however, such as death or severe illness, there is an expected exchange of food in the community. The other time this happens is when the gardens begin to produce and foodstuffs are exchanged along kinship and friendship lines (support groups). These food exchanges comprise the only supplemental source of food in households. Such ritualistic exchanges symbolize the strength of social relationships and also function as redistribution mechanisms. Some food is given as charity by the churches, and the Food Stamp Program helps lower income families; indeed, many households in Coberly would be unable to purchase sufficient food without this program. Households in which the parent(s) work find it difficult to "get to the store." In these households children are often sent to purchase the food for supper. The woman of the household generally cooks the meals, sometimes with the help of the older children (usually female). A few of the upper income families have cooks who purchase the ingredients for meals, which are, however, generally planned by the woman of the household.

Food has important meanings for the people of Coberly. Certain foods are symbols of social class and health status. About half of the Blacks and Whites of Coberly eat specific foods to enhance their health. The most desired part of their diet is vegetables (such as greens and carrots to put vitamins in the blood), with "greens" (e.g., turnip greens) more frequently mentioned by lower income people. Though Whites feel meats are important in the diet, Blacks discussed it more frequently as an item they feel should be a part of their diet.

Additional foods Coberlians eat are cereals, juices, salads, fruits, protein, liver, salty foods, starchy foods, fried foods, and "old timey foods." Women, by far, name more foods than men. Indeed, over half of the men do not feel that their diet could affect their health significantly. Besides vegetables (often cooked with fat), the men feel that fried foods and beef are good for health. Women feel that eating breakfast and at least one other "balanced meal" is important. Several of the older women said they had learned about a balanced diet at the senior citizens' center. Over and over again, the women, both Black and White, stated that eating a variety of foods is important for diet and health. Some of the foods they believe are good for one's health are actually not, according to modern medicine. The problem of diet among the people of Coberly is not, however, so much the kinds of food as how they are cooked and the quantity of food consumed. Vegetables are prepared "Southern style"; i.e., cooked until mushy with a great deal of salt and frequently with pork or fatback. Often this is the only meat the poor have at a meal; it is the cheapest available in the grocery stores.

Avoiding foods that may be harmful to one's health is a behavior that is not especially familiar to the people of Coberly, especially to Blacks and younger men. About 50 percent do not avoid any foods for health purposes. Women, however, discussed a wide range of foods they avoid to improve or maintain their health. And, since it is the woman who is most often responsible for the meals served in the household, men generally must rely on the choices their wives or mothers make. Women say they try to avoid greasy foods, fried foods, sweets, and pork but that they find it difficult, if not impossible. Very few discussed salt or salty foods and no one reported avoiding foods with preservatives or artificial flavorings. Males who did discuss avoiding foods (mostly those over 50 years old) mentioned avoiding pork more frequently than fatty foods in general or sweets.

A distinctive pattern emerged between Blacks and Whites in Coberly: Whites named a wider variety of foods they avoided than Blacks. Those Whites who are aware of the relationship between food and health and act upon this awareness discussed the dangers of eating greasy foods, pork and sweets, but also reported avoiding butter, white bread, junk food, salt and salty meats, onions, liver and foods high in cholesterol. Blacks concentrated simply on greasy foods, pork and sugar/sweets. Overall, the avoidance of certain foods and the eating of specific other foods for health is a behavior of middle income Whites and older Blacks who have "high blood" problems. Many of the households of both Blacks and Whites, moreover, had a variety of the foods the respondents said they knew they should avoid. When questioned about this discrepancy, they often said it is difficult to change one's eating habits or that someone else in the house had purchased the items. Even though they know they should not eat certain foods, "they taste good" or "they are the only foods we can afford."

One health management pattern that emerged among both Blacks and the white elderly was knowledge of the relationship between food and bowel movement. While many of the elderly take laxatives regularly, they often reported that their doctor had suggested eating specific foods instead. They are attempting to comply by eating cereals with bran or other fiber, and apples, and by drinking fruit juices. They would show these products to me frequently and said that television advertisements convinced them that the doctors were right in suggesting these foods. Regularity is a major concern of the elderly and when the foodstuff or liquids do not work they still resort to laxatives, generally Exlax, Feenamint or Epsom Salts.

Exercise

A form of healthful activity engaged in by about half of the people of Coberly is exercise. Whites consciously exercise for health much more than do Blacks. Most upper income Whites exercise on a weekly basis, and their activities are different from those of poor Whites and Blacks. For example, one middle income White exercises on a trampoline and plays tennis, while another "bicycles and plays tennis and golf at the country club." Besides walking, biking and yard work, other activities upper and middle income Whites frequently engage in are exercise classes, playing ball with the kids, running, exercises at home, swimming and housework. Most of them engage in multiple activities and do so on a regular basis. Lower income Whites exclusively work, walk or do housework for exercise.

Similarly, when asked what forms of exercises they engage in regularly, Blacks overwhelmingly named working; i.e., the physical activities they normally engage in on the job. Other activities they think of as exercise are yardwork, gardening, and walking. Only one person rode a bicycle or did specific exercises at home (the treatment prescribed by the doctor for a leg injury). Typically, people would report, "I walk to town sometimes"; "working in the yard"; "my job requires exercise"; or "I get exercise around the yard and at work" as exercise activities. Blacks infrequently discussed multiple forms of exercise.

Distinctive patterns emerged between men and women, and particularly between women of different economic levels. White middle income women participate in activities that can be categorized as recreational, such as swimming, tennis or bicycle riding, or have an exercise routine based on books or manuals they read. Likewise, white men get exercise through recreation—playing ball and tennis—or through their hobbies, such as gardening. Lower income white women participate in activities similar to those of black women; i.e., housework is their only form of exercise. In general, however, women reported more activities and more multiple activities than men, who overwhelmingly think that work is their basic exercise. A frequent topic of conversation in households was the interest young people have in exercise. Their sons and daughters exercise more frequently than the adults, a valuable lesson they have learned at school. Knowledge of exercise is not generally transmitted from parents to children and, in general, except in middle income families, Coberlians make very little connection between exercise and health.

Unlike in urban areas, one does not observe people running, riding bicycles or walking in the mornings or afternoons in Coberly. These activities are not considered family activities. People do not walk to shop or visit. They ride in cars. Riding "somewhere" is generally a group activity even if it takes only a few minutes. "Going to town" or "going to see Aunt Sue" in the car, even though it may be a journey of only two or three blocks, is an important family activity and most of the time, people drive from one part of town to another (3 or 4 blocks) rather than walk.

Tobacco Use

The people of Coberly use tobacco extensively—over two-thirds of the population—and, with the exception of upper income people, are not readily concerned about its effect on their health. The amount of tobacco consumed on a daily basis is higher among Blacks than Whites. Almost 68 percent of black women use tobacco, compared with 42 percent of white women, the group which uses tobacco the least. Men, both black and white, use tobacco more frequently than women, and they do so in greater quantities. We found no significant differences among different income and age levels.

We did discover differences between Blacks and Whites in terms of the types of tobacco they use, however. Overall, Blacks use multiple types of tobacco in conjunction with one another during the day. In addition to smoking cigarettes, Blacks chew tobacco, dip snuff and smoke cigars, while Whites primarily smoke cigarettes or pipes, with a very small percentage chewing tobacco or dipping snuff. One woman, who chews and smokes, continually asks God to forgive her if it is, indeed, a sin. She believes it relieves stress and that she would be ill without the habit. In fact, most Coberlians feel that smoking is a habit that, if abandoned, would create more health problems than it would cure. Some of these problems are "nerves," overeating and sleeplessness.

The quantity of tobacco used in Coberly is very high. People who smoke cigarettes average over a pack per day, with some reporting up to five packs in a twenty-four hour period and others only four or five cigarettes a day. Several people dip snuff "all the time" while others dip only after meals. Most Coberlians who dip snuff do so two to three times per day on the average. Similarly, a few people chew tobacco all day, although the majority use 'a few (3-5) pinches two or three times a day, often after every meal. Tobacco use is normally associated with the intake of food; people talked about tobacco use as if they were talking medicines: "three or four times a day or half a pack a day and after each meal." Most believe that chewing and dipping tobacco is healthier than smoking cigarettes and say that these behaviors keep them from smoking too much. Overall, Coberlians classified tobacco use as health promoting rather than as disease causing. Their knowledge of healthy behavior (such as exercise and a good diet) does not extend to tobacco use.

Colds and Flu

Colds and flu are chronic problems for the people of Coberly, as they are for the American public in general. Since they are maladies most people have to contend with, we asked specific questions about the preventive behaviors that circumvent colds and flu. Not only did this questioning elicit information about their beliefs and behaviors about preventive measures in general, but their answers also gave us a clue to the resources through which they acquire their knowledge about preventive medicines.

To begin with, colds are associated with one season—winter—and about 30 percent of the people interviewed feel that they can partially if not altogether prevent colds in the winter. The most frequent preventive measures among Blacks and Whites are taking Vitamin C and staying warm. Blacks talked about staying out of the rain, staying dry, wearing warm clothing, drinking a lot of liquids, eating fruit, and taking castor oil and aspirin as deterrents. Only one had taken a flu shot. Whites' repertoire is smaller, and most white men feel that one cannot prevent colds, so they refuse to engage in any preventive behavior unless their wives or mothers force them to. Women enjoy talking about giving medicines to their husbands and/or sons to prevent colds.

Likewise, it is the women of Coberly who take care of household members when they get colds. Although men said they take aspirin and over-the-counter drugs, it is the women who purchase medicine and give the men and children advice about health behavior in general; the treatment of colds thus exemplifies general household behavior patterns. Over-the-counter medicines are most frequently used for colds; aspirin, Tylenol, Nyquil, Alka-Seltzer Plus, and Contact are taken in combination with the drinking of juices and other liquids and resting more for a few days. In addition, Coberlians use home remedies for colds and the flu, the most common being mixtures of whiskey, honey and lemon juice and/or yellow root and pomegranate tea. One woman boils needles from the east side of a pine tree, strains the mixture and drinks the liquid. Often home remedies are mixed with over-the-counter medicines. When this occurs, the dosage of over-the-counter cold medicines is reduced. The general pattern for treating the flu and colds, then, is to rely on medicine from drug stores and, especially for people in the lower income bracket, to combine them with home remedies. If these behaviors are not effective in a few days or weeks, a doctor is sometimes consulted as a last resort. Lower income people rarely said they see a doctor for colds and the flu. They just "wait it out" and use the traditional approaches to such maladies.

Care for the Elderly

Care for the elderly is rapidly becoming a national problem. The fastest growing age group in the United States is people over 65 years of age; in fact, the over 75 years group has grown by more than 37 percent in the last ten years. This "graying of America" is perceived as no more of a problem now than it has been in the past by most people in Coberly. Coberlians have always "taken care of their old people" and continue to do so in much the same way they have in the past. Of course, the federal government has, since 1965 with the passage of Medicare, helped with the health problems of the elderly, although many people did not take advantage of Medicare or Medicaid for years after that date. They were either unaware of these programs' existence or did not know how to use the system. Only within the last decade have the people of Coberly learned to use Medicare with any frequency, allowing them to use the health care system for some of their health problems. Most of the elderly in Coberly receive their income from Social Security benefits. Most men are retired from jobs such as farming or laboring, while most women have been housewives all their lives. Some of their jobs did not pay into Social Security, however, and these senior citizens cannot receive benefits. Consequently, the main problem of care for the elderly is how to link into two systems: the governmental system and the family system.

The Older American Act of 1978 calls for the planning of social service programs for senior citizens. States have been delegated the power to delineate the needs of the elderly and to implement programs to meet these needs. In Coberly, the main need so far is considered to be food. Therefore, the major emphasis of the senior citizens' center was nutrition education. Since the time of this study, however, as mentioned earlier, this center has been closed. Federal funding for health problems of the elderly has been cut recently and those programs in existence are now biased toward acute episodes even though, as we found in Coberly, a majority of the elderly suffer from chronic diseases. Some of these diseases are debilitating to the point that persons cannot take care of themselves and require outside assistance, either from relatives/friends or from governmental or private resources (such as a home for the elderly). Cober County has a "rest home" which is normally filled to over 90 percent of its capacity. This resource, however, is used as a "last resort" by the people of the county, only after all other alternatives for caring for the elderly have been exhausted. Several people have given up their jobs in order to stay home and take care of an elderly person in the family, a loss to the work force and a loss to the household income. These are sacrifices, however, that most people feel must be made in order to fulfill their obligations to their families and keep from having to place an elderly member in the nursing home.

Most black and white elderly in Coberly live with or near relatives, usually a son, daughter, brother or sister. Younger members of the family, including the children, take responsibility for caring for them during certain times of the day or week. This situation occurs when an elderly person cannot live by himself/herself because of illness or the death of a spouse. Until one of these events occurs, the elderly of Coberly do live by themselves. Almost every elderly person, black or white, lives near relatives, often "next door," or "across the street." One person said he bought a trailer and placed it behind his house so his mother could live close to him. Most elderly people, however, have brothers, sisters, sons, daughters or cousins who live in their community.

These family members and occasionally a neighbor take the major responsibility for their elderly relatives. They drive them to church, to the doctor, to family gatherings and to the grocery store. With the exception of these occasions, though, we found that many elderly are usually alone. They feel isolated and lonely, making for rather serious mental health problems—none of which were reported by the people themselves, only by the health personnel in the town. Loneliness is a condition the elderly accept as part of the process of getting old. Their relationships change and isolate them more from their families and friends. Each individual must accept that this is a "normal" process and that it is up to him or her to cope with the feelings. Greenhouse reports that in Hopewell, "Emotional self-sufficiency is supposed to grow with age" (1986:70). Similarly, in Coberly the elderly do not perceive loneliness as a problem to talk about or report to an anthropologist. I found, as did Kivett and Scott (1979) in North Carolina, that mental health problems are underreported and that the elderly want to remain independent for as long as possible, although most are dependent on others for transportation and shopping.

The health problems of the elderly in Coberly reflect the well health patterns of the community and the general differential patterns between Blacks and Whites. The most frequent health problems of the black elderly are "high blood," arthritis and diabetes (often self-diagnosed). Several had experienced strokes or heart-related problems. For example, an elderly man and woman (husband and wife) said that they had "weak hearts" and "high blood." In addition, the wife has diabetes and they both have arthritis. In spite of these multiple chronic problems, they live alone, grow most of the vegetables they eat, and rely on their son to take them into town (the square) to purchase the essentials for daily living and to visit the doctor if necessary. Both have a variety of prescription medicines in their house, but they reported they do not take them regularly, only when they feel "bad." They also told us that they fear the young people who pass their house every day who, according to them, harass them frequently.

The white elderly also have multiple chronic problems and reported a wider range of illnesses than Blacks. The most frequent problems are those related to heart malfunctions. A stroke has been experienced by twice as many Whites as Blacks. Almost all Blacks and Whites have arthritis, while Whites have experienced cancer more frequently than Blacks. Additional problems of the white elderly are arteriosclerosis (hardening of the arteries), phlebitis, and cirrhosis of the liver, none of which were reported by Blacks. All, however, discussed the problems of "getting old," such as not being able to see or hear well and slowness in recovering from colds.

There are additional health problems reported by the health personnel that, interestingly, were not mentioned by the people themselves. While they felt that the most serious overall health problems all related to eating habits, these professionals specifically pointed out hypertension, obesity, arthritis and isolation as problems for Blacks and arthritis, loneliness and depression for Whites. None of our respondents talked about depression as a problem for them or members of their household.

We found, contrary to what health personnel reported, that isolation and consequent depression are problems among Blacks as well as Whites. Many of the elderly of Coberly are alone, and many do not eat nutritious diets, which compounds their problems. Although some are aware of the foods they should avoid, most are not, and even if they are told, they either find it too difficult to change their diet or they cannot afford to purchase more nutritious foods.

Because the regional planning commission was able to document these problems, funds for the senior citizens' center were acquired for the specific purpose of serving meals to the elderly. In addition, though, the center helped alleviate the feelings of loneliness and isolation that are problems for many other people. Emphasis was placed on information about nutrition; other programs focused on the problems of living alone, a variety of arts and crafts, and reducing energy costs. People strong enough to ride were picked up daily by a van, taken to the center around 10 a.m. and returned to their homes by mid-afternoon. Governmental regulations placed time and mileage constraints on the program, however, which prevented some elderly who lived too far away from participating in the program.

We observed the behavior of the elderly in the senior citizens' center over a four-month period. The seating arrangements and patterns of interactions there reflected the general ethnic patterns in the community. Very rarely did Blacks and Whites interact; furthermore, males and females usually segregated themselves in separate rooms. The men (mostly black) sat in the room with a television set and rarely talked to one another. The white women congregated around a table and exchanged gossip about people in the town or about their families. The black women did the same, but separately. Topics discussed frequently by both groups were their problems and death. Often, death was discussed in a semi-joking manner. The director of the center felt that the elderly were preoccupied with the topic and often became morbid in conversations. One woman frequently said, "you never know when you put your shoes on in the morning, you never know who will take them off at night." Their discussions about health generally focused on comparing problems, medicines and treatment prescribed by their doctors.

Older people came to the center for a variety of reasons, but the main one seemed to be to get a meal. Most said that they were not interested in the educational programs, but that the food they got once a day was worth participating in the other activities. Others felt that, in addition to the meal, the opportunity to get out of the house was incentive enough to participate in the center's activities. Several said that they sometimes went days without talking to anyone (except via telephone). Finally, some participated in the center's programs more during the winter than during the summer because they could stay warm during the hours at the center. They could not afford to heat their houses properly due to high heating bills or to their inability to keep a fire going all day.

Since this program was county-wide, we were able to discover the overall patterns of the elderly outside Coberly as well. A large majority of participants in the center were women, some of whom lived alone and whose only daily contact was with the people in the center. These women were more isolated and often lived alone since, especially among Blacks, men die much earlier than women. These rural women often had serious problems with depression, dietary patterns and chronic health problems. Such women living alone typically have little money and often very little social contact, especially if their children live far away.

The form of intervention into the problems of the elderly by programs such as this is important. We found that this program was not effective in changing health behavior. While the elderly who went to the center were exposed to nutritional information, they did not put into practice the suggested changes in cooking and eating habits. Intervention strategies were not framed in terms of their system but in terms of the medical system. One way this problem could have been avoided would have been, for example, to have the senior citizens cook their own food at the center rather than having the meals brought in hot boxes from a city 60 miles away. In addition, home visits would have alleviated some of their loneliness and isolation. Although intervention strategies will be discussed in Chapter 7, here several techniques which could be used to reach these poor elderly might be mentioned. Kivett and Scott state that "older rural adults need viable supports available to them that will keep important aspects of their life style intact while improving the overall quality of life" (1979:59). Indeed there is "a high extent of interrelationship between the physical, social and environmental characteristics of older adults living in rural isolated areas . . . " (1979:58). There is a need for intervention in several important areas such as transportation, decentralization of health centers for multiphasic screening, effective emergency transportation, quality housing, and services and programs that facilitate independence and prevent or delay institutionalization.

Management and Perceptions of Mental Health Problems

Distinguishing physical from mental health is a difficult task. Indeed, separating the mind from the body is dangerous conceptually, and when applied to actual behavior and illnesses it can be very misleading. Although there is a scarcity of data on rural areas (Cross and Dengerink 1982), many mental health problems occur, it would appear, because of the tremendous changes in the economic, social and political structures of rural communities. Rural communities have experienced economic decline, a decrease in employment opportunities, a lack of recreational activities and an acute level of poverty, all of which lower the quality of life. People lose control of their communities and in many ways, control of their lives, often with serious psychological repercussions. In many cases, however, the psychological problems of people in rural areas are managed by the community itself.

Studies in rural areas have provided detailed data on the management of mental health in traditional communities. From these studies it becomes clear that there is a greater acceptance of behavior labeled "abnormal" in rural areas. The boundaries of such behavior may be more open than in urban areas, and once people go beyond those boundaries, if they are not harmful to themselves or to others, they are often given roles in the community which allow them to continue to function. In the rural South, mental health is considered the domain of institutions such as the family or religion; people refrain from linking to public institutions such as mental health clinics. Only the most desperate, who lack traditional social support or who are destructive to the community, will be forced by their families or by public officials to use public mental health facilities.

Since family relationships and roles are not negotiable and cannot change, seeking help from mental health workers is the antithesis of the people of Coberly's beliefs about family and community. As Greenhouse reports " . . . individual roles are seen as fixed in their personalities, which are unalterable except by God" (1986:53). If there are problems one renegotiates with oneself and with God, but not by changing the roles within a family as set down by God. Again, Greenhouse has captured this process in a neighboring community of Hopewell. She states, "All conflict immediately becomes inner conflict first and foremost. The only appropriate remedies are interior. People deal with conflict by internalizing it" (1986:153). The church plays an important role by providing the inner resources the people need to deal with problems of role conflict and mental disorders. Linking to systems outside the family and church negates Coberlians' worldview.

In Coberly, mental health problems are therefore either neglected or dealt with by families and/or the community. Coberlians discussed with us the individuals in the town who often "acted strange" but "did not hurt anyone," like the man who sometimes wears his mother's clothes downtown. He lives outside the city limits and several times a year dresses in women's clothes. He spends part of the day in town shopping, talking to people and eating. No one calls any kind of authority; they just tolerate this abberant behavior. Another person, a white woman about 55 years old, and from an upper income family, is known to be on drugs. She frequently drives into town on the wrong side of the road and sometimes sits in the passenger's seat. Coberlians "just get out of her way" since she does not hurt anyone.

Only when persons are harmful to themselves, to their families, or to the community are they taken, most often by family members, to the doctor or to the hospital for help. Consequently, the number of cases admitted to mental health facilities is very low. Overall, rural usage of Community

Mental Health Centers (CMHC) is less frequent for all racial/ethnic groups than usage in urban centers. As in most rural areas, there are no "crisis intervention" services in Coberly; crises are taken care of by the family.

Coberlians were asked for their ideas about alcoholism, drugs, family abuse and general mental problems. Seventy percent of them feel that alcoholism is the major health problem among all ages, while 78 percent feel that drug usage is the major problem among the young people in the community. In responding to the question "What causes these problems?", most believe that they result from lack of activities such as recreation or work. Other answers include "Because they want to get high," and "Never been taught right." More Blacks than Whites stated that alcohol and drug usage are ways of trying to deal with personal problems and pressures, frequently involving not having enough money or not having a job. Alcohol and drugs allow people to relax and forget their problems for awhile. Many adults think that young people do not have enough to do after school and that those who are out of school often cannot find steady jobs. Thus, they become bored and, yielding to peer pressure, they begin using drugs or drinking. Overall, Blacks have a higher awareness of drug usage in the community than do Whites.

The Whites of Coberly talked about "stress" rather than "pressure" and believe that stress is caused by economic problems, loneliness, personal difficulties, and family problems. One person said that "much of drinking is caused by Southern culture, with its strict moral code and intense family relationships." Whites, but not Blacks mentioned "insecurity," "inhibition," and "immaturity" as reasons for drinking but, like Blacks, they feel that boredom and peer pressure also cause people to drink. Whites tend to equate alcohol and drug usage, but the factors they believe cause drug abuse extend beyond social problems to include psychological problems such as "depression" and the need for an "escape mechanism." Several feel that smoking pot is better than drinking and, if done in moderation, is not harmful. A few even think it should be legalized.

Coberlians' beliefs about intervention mechanisms for alcoholism or problem drinking integrate with their beliefs about intervention for physical health problems (Chapter 5) and with their worldview in general—it is up to the individual to heal himself/herself. The individual is not necessarily blamed for a drug or drinking problem, but it is thought that the individual is responsible for overcoming these problems. He/she can, however, be aided by God, the minister, and in some cases other outside help such as clinics or special organizations. For alcoholism, a majority of Whites discussed the need for a local chapter of Alcoholics Anonymous and a mental health clinic. While Blacks did not mention AA, they did express a need for "some kind of office or person who can deal with this problem." Blacks discussed a need for a drug clinic and counseling in schools, while Whites emphasized the existing facilites and professional personnel in neighboring towns. Some people of Coberly are beginning to see a need to link with outside services. Others feel that if the conditions in the communtiy were changed, these problems would subside. For example, several Blacks mentioned that if their living situation were better, not as many Blacks would drink. Both Blacks and Whites feel that better law enforcement would help alleviate drug problems in the community. Many Blacks and Whites also feel that in addition to professional help, God, the minister, and family support can help with drug abuse problems and, as with drinking problems, drug usage would be lessened if young people had "more to do" in the town. Interestingly, only one White said that doctors can help people with these problems.

We asked the people of Coberly about child abuse and family violence, a question that made the respondents very uncomfortable, much more so than the question on alcohol and drug abuse. Twenty-nine percent were aware of such behavior either in their family or in the community. They have no ideas about how to stop or intervene in such aberrant behavior, however. A majority of the Blacks who did respond to this question feel that legal intervention combined with parental counseling is the best strategy. They believe that abusive parents were raised in the same sort of environment, meaning the parents had probably undergone abuse themselves. When pressed to give a reason for this, several said, "It is because of the pressures of living." No Whites discussed legal solutions in terms of calling the authorities during an actual violent event, but some did stress taking the children away from the parents. Many feel that "These are family problems," and that no one should get involved. Upper income people (all White) believe it is a problem of "the poor and black." Generally, people are either unaware of child abuse and family violence or, even with our probing, were reluctant to discuss such problems. We did, however, hear about numerous events that convinced us that child and family abuse is a problem in the community.

People were less reluctant to discuss general mental health problems. Only 50 percent think that there are people in Coberly with such problems. We framed our questions in terms of "mental problems" and some of our prodding including the using of hypothetical situations. For example, the question "If you thought someone you knew was having some mental problems, what would you do?" elicited varied responses from Blacks and Whites. A few Whites discussed available facilities, professional personnel in nearby towns and the family doctor. Most said that they would advise the person to rely on the Lord, the minister and his/her family. Indeed, one person stated, "Get to the root of the problem; use all resources including the church, rehabilitation services and social networks." Others would talk to the person and tell him or her that if he/she "does the right thing," he/she will have nothing to fear. Only one Black mentioned a clinic or institution, while most named the minister, the family and a doctor (not a family doctor). Blacks are generally unaware of situations in which mental health facilities were used. If they have not experienced a specific event, they are also generally unaware of the available resources located outside the county. They often generalize for the entire population, however, based on knowledge of one event. Suicide was discussed at social gatherings in the homes but usually briefly and with an air of secrecy. There has been only one suicide in Coberly during the past ten years.

When asked directly where people can get help for mental health problems, only four percent of the people of Coberly mentioned a mental health facility. As previously stated, most believe that it is up to the affected person, his/her family, God, or the law. While Whites frequently mentioned counseling, over 80 percent of the poor are unaware of the public resources for mental health intervention. A majority of Blacks said that the family takes care of the mentally ill. Likewise, Whites said that the family is the key resource for caring for the mentally ill, with upper income people frequently mentioning the hospital and/or clinic in the district. A few said they would consult a doctor or a psychologist. No one discussed or had consulted a nurse, a social worker, the primary health care clinic, or the public health clinic for mental health problems.

In an attempt to discover the basis on which Coberlians decide whether or not a person is mentally ill, we asked how they recognized a mental problem in a person. As expected, most responded in terms of behavioral changes. A common response was, "they act crazy, or strange, not normal." Several Blacks reported that "talking to oneself is a sure sign of mental problems." Likewise, a person who "looks worried or discontented or confused" is possibly mentally ill. Although a "mental problem" is a category distinct from drinking or drug abuse, a majority of Blacks related such problems to "drinking too much." Likewise, Whites associated mental health problems with drinking, but middle and upper income Whites draw from a wider vocabulary to describe the behavior of people with mental problems. Acting anxious, discontented, irrational, depressed, suicidal, and psychotic are typical descriptions used by those Whites.

Can people recover from mental problems? The majority (52 percent) of the people of Coberly think not; once a person has such a problem, he/she can never be fully "cured." Almost 40 percent of Blacks believe that "it is up to the Lord," for a person to recover and even then it depends on the severity of the problem. Many told us stories about a member of their family or a friend who had "a nervous breakdown," or "a mental condition," who never really became "normal." They would be taken away for a while and when they returned would be "right" for a time but would then often would "act crazy" again. Whites believe that the chance of recovery depends on the cause of the illness and the person. If mental problems are inherited, then no one can help. If mental problems are caused by social stresses, then the person "might can be cured" if he/she receives the "right treatment." For example, one person said that "it can be cured if caught in the right stage or if it is a mild case," while another stated, "if they get treated properly with the right treatment and love and care." It was also thought that a cure could result from "the right treatment and medication." Often, "the right treatment" referred to the use of drugs or to psychological help, especially for upper income people. For other groups, it referred to listening to the Lord, to the advice of family members and to oneself.

Social changes and inner changes involve changing a person's beliefs and behaviors to conform to community values and norms. In Coberly, people who have mental problems ultimately must deal with themselves and with their relationships to their families, their community and God. The cases of David and Ann illustrate that family and community are, in Coberly, the crucial links for the individual in his/her response to and management of mental health problems.

The Case of David

A white man who has been married for 14 years and has 3 children, David was 35 years old when he began to go out with other women and drink in public. He worked at a factory in a nearby town and, at the time he changed his ways, was at high risk of being laid off. For the previous 14 years, he had refrained from participating in community activities, including going to church. He was, however, considered to be a "good family man" in that he provided for his wife and children, did not break the law, hung out with his men friends only occasionally and took care of his mother who lived alone outside Coberly. He did not get along well with his brother, who had moved to Magnolia and who did not help David with their mother. About a year before this study, David's mother got sick and he was told that he might lose his job. At that point, his public and private behavior changed. He didn't get along with his wife, and their relationship was estranged to the point that he began being seen with other, younger women. He also began to drink and was picked up by the police several times for drunken driving. Such behavior continued for several months until one day he was driving down a road late one night and wrecked his car. When he woke up in the hospital, he was frightened about the fact that he could have died. His family was there by his bedside, as was the preacher from the church his wife and children attended. After going home and having to stay in bed for two weeks, he realized that the Lord was giving him a sign to change his ways and become a good father, husband and son again.

When he was able to walk, he joined the church and decided that God had given him another chance in life. He had never thought of utilizing the mental health resources in the area while he was experiencing the stress of work and family problems. This was not an option in his worldview. "That is where crazy people go" was David's response to using mental health facilities.

The Case of Ann

Ann is a 58-year-old black woman who has seven children and 12 grandchildren. She lives with two of her daughters and their four children. Her husband left years ago to work in the North and sent money for awhile. He rarely contacts her or the children anymore. About four years ago Ann began to lose her temper more frequently than usual and, as time went on, she would get in fights with neighbors, shopkeepers, and family members. It did not appear that anything had changed in her life except that she had "gone through the change awhile back" and one of her daughters had lost her job. One of her granddaughters was also having a hard time in school; she had not made the cheerleading team and was not doing well in math and English. One day Ann caused a scene at the grocery store and would not leave the store until the owner gave her the ten dollars she said he owed her. The police were called, and forcibly put Ann in a police car and took her home. At this point, family and friends began to talk to her about her outbursts. Her daughter talked to their preacher and their doctor, neither of whom suggested that she go to the mental health clinic. The doctor thought it was a "middle life crisis" that would pass, and the preacher suggested that she pray more often to God for his guidance. Ann began to drink more than usual and at the same time, to go to church more. Her family now stays with her and will not let her go out by herself, and they have an elderly woman who is thought to "know about these things" come to see her to talk about her problems. She is kept out of public places as much as possible, and at home she is cared for by her children and grandchildren.

These cases demonstrate that rural people such as those in Coberly underutilize mental health services for many reasons, even though stresses in this environment occur no less frequently than in urban areas. In fact, the stereotype of the tranquil life in rural areas is a myth. Life there is just as stressful and is often more so in situations of rapid social change or of high unemployment. Under these conditions, people often have difficulty, as did David and Ann, coping with their social surroundings. Only in extreme cases, though, will they link voluntarily to the mental health system. The reasons for this underutilization of mental health facilities include: (1) the population's lack of knowledge about the existence of services and/or about the types of services available; (2) lack of referrals to mental health facilities; (3) available services which do not meet the needs or expectations of the target population; (4) people's perception of mental health facilities as being a hostile environment and as representing the dominant group's institutions; (5) problems with transportation which restrict access; (6) the perception of mental health as not separate from physical health, and thus the seeking of mental health care from medical practitioners; (7) cultural valuation of mental health or stigmas against mental illness preventing individuals from seeking services; and (8) assistance for mental health problems being sought from alternative sources, such as family members, religious leaders, traditional healers, teachers, or respected community leaders. All of these factors operate in Coberly. Besides the stigma associated with mental illness, there is the problem of the ideological and social structures of the community, which are in conflict with the concepts of mental health service delivery accepted by professionals (Wagenfeld and Wagenfeld 1981).

Just how do people manage their mental health problems if not through institutional means? The answer is that most of them manage through traditional institutions (family, church) or wind up in the criminal justice system and/or with an alcohol or drug problem. In 1974, Rosen found that utilization rates in rural areas are lower than in urban areas for mental health facilities, and attributed this situation to social attitudes, greater tolerance of deviant behavior, appropriateness of service and accessibility and, in the Southern states, a feeling of disdain toward public health facilities. These factors appear to apply to mental health facilities in Coberly, where most people feel that mental health problems are family and community problems that should be solved within the community. Although the people of Coberly do not feel disdain for health clinics, they do have misgivings about using mental health resources unless the services are for alcohol or drug abuse.

Summary

In this chapter, decision making about health promotion and mental health has been placed within the context of community and family in Coberly. The medical system in rural communities is superimposed on cultural and social systems and, in many cases, the fit is imperfect. Linkages in the structure of the health care system can be rationally planned by policy-makers but the linkages that make a difference in the system's fulfilling its purpose are made by the people in rural communities.

The most important social institutions for the people of Coberly in their responses to illness (whether physical or mental) are the family and the community. Most people have a rather closed worldview, with their identity and security coming from their interactions with family, friends and the workplace. Only some of the upper income Whites have a worldview that opens to include alternative lifestyles beyond Cober County or the surrounding area. Health, then, is managed within these social institutions and linkages to the health system, to a large extent, depend on people's stage in the life cycle, their ethnic background and income level. Again in this chapter we have seen that considering the heterogeneity of a population is crucial in anticipating how people in a community will link to the health system. Another factor in understanding and predicting decisions about health care is the belief system that negotiates the symbols which provide meaning—in this case, to the people of Coberly. This will be explored in the next chapter.

5

Popular Medicine, Health Beliefs, and Cultural Models

We have seen that the people of Coberly are eclectic in their health behavior. Their patterns of illness behavior, health promotion behavior, and utilization of health facilities reflect their beliefs, connecting their health system to the cultural and social systems that make sense of their lives. Their beliefs about the causes of illness, the treatment of illnesses, the place of family and God in their lives, the effectiveness of doctors and their medicines, and the effectiveness of traditional healers and home remedies set the parameters for their behavior. These beliefs constitute their health cultural model; such models, according to Quinn and Holland are the basis of action of people (1987).

Coberlians' cultural model extends the biomedical model of health to include alternative health behaviors which they feel complement the scientific approach. A major aspect of their health model is the idea of self-involvement: the belief that one can to some extent control his/her health status. People not only cause themselves to become ill, but can also heal themselves with the "right beliefs" and proper behaviors. Furthermore, Coberlians believe that the affected person should be actively engaged in the illness and health process. Self-help and independent decision making are thus integral parts of their health cultural model which is reflected in their health behavior.

Popular Medicines in the South

An estimated 80–90 percent of health problems in Coberly are handled using forms of popular medicine—home remedies and other self-help behaviors—within the family/household context, or using specialists outside the biomedical model (Kleinman 1977). Popular medicine in the South is an ongoing system of health resources used by many people in the region as one option for help during times of medical crises. Although we do not have exact statistics on the distribution and frequency of the use of popular medicine, we do know that it is widespread, particularly among the poor in both rural and urban areas. Popular medicine is defined as a cultural system distinct from the biomedical cultural system, and includes the use of herbs, roots, over-the-counter drugs and healing specialists. It is a viable system based on a theory that integrates knowledge of scientific medicine with traditional knowledge.

Popular medicine is utilized for chronic problems more frequently than for acute ones, by both Blacks and Whites, men and women. Women are most often turned to for help in the health-seeking process; men, however, may also be healers. There are few ethnic boundaries in utilizing healers in the South. Weidman (1978) reports that in choosing a healer, the power of the healer is more important to the client than his/her ethnic background. Most of the people who use healers are poor, although the use of popular medicine is not limited to poor people. Indeed, most people use some kind of popular medicine in addition to scientific medicine (Hill and Mathews 1981).

Illnesses treated in the home generally exhibit familiar symptoms and do not seriously physically incapacitate the victim. Most home remedies are easily available animal products (e.g., milk, fat, bones), chemical or mineral substances (e.g., sulphur, ashes, vinegar, sugar, turpentine) or plants (e.g., yellow root, tree bark, sassafras). A variety of these substances is kept in the home for use in treating colds, indigestion, burns, sores, sore throats, fevers, headaches, and general aches and pains. Plants are generally administered in the form of teas. Knowledge of the use of these remedies is widespread, and the substance may vary depending on the health problem, though the behavior stays intact. For example, many remedies used in the home are over-the-counter medicines whose repertoire keeps shifting. More recently, there seems to be an increasing reliance on medicines advertised in the media, or "media medicine." There are thus remedies that have been used for years to which are added new ones advertised by drug companies. The new medications are incorporated into people's health beliefs and behaviors. Healers will often combine them with more traditional roots or herbs in their treatment of illness. For example, a healer often prescribes Pepto-Bismol mixed with whiskey for the "shakes."

There are several types of traditional healers in the rural and urban South. They are referred to by a variety of names: hoodoo doctor, voodoo doctor, herb doctor, root doctor and conjurer, for example. The practice of voodoo medicine is now concentrated on the coasts of Georgia and

South Carolina and in Southern Louisiana, although its influence has survived in other areas with large numbers of Blacks. Some voodoo specialists have reputations that span several hundred miles, and people travel considerable distances to see them and be healed (Jordan 1975, Snow 1978, 1979). Indeed, Jordan (1975) points out that voodoo is a coherent system that incorporates many elements, including those of biomedicine.

Some healers are believed to be particularly competent to treat specific problems. For example, there are specialists who "talk the fire out of burns," "stop bleeding," "cure the thrash" and "conjure warts" (Hill 1973, 1976). Root doctors are often used for "high blood" or "low blood" and other ailments such as headaches, tiredness or itching. They may heal with herbal remedies (a natural condition) or with "rootworks" (an unnatural condition). They are frequently consulted by people who participate in the folk and the scientific medical systems (Murphree 1976; Hall and Bourne 1973; Snell 1967; Tingling 1967; Wintrob 1973; Cappanari et al. 1975; Quinn and Mathews n.d.). Other healers have the knowledge and ability to rid the body of general aches and pains and relieve mental stress.

People use these specialists for symptoms such as headaches, backaches, occasional loss of memory, tiredness, thinking about a particular subject or person too much and sexual impotency. Folk specialists diagnose such cases as overwork, "nerves" or worry. They don't strictly separate the problems of their clients into mental and physical problems. The healers generally spend a great deal of time with their clients obtaining knowledge about their social life or religious life before making a diagnosis and recommending treatment. Clients are consequently treated on physical, psychological and social levels simultaneously. Through ritually using roots and herbs, recommending dietary change, using popular medicines, reading passages from the Bible, and offering counseling, the healer attempts to restore a balance in the patient's life.

Folk beliefs about health are widely shared by people who practice folk medicine. Obviously, folk concepts of disease and illness involve a broader conceptual framework than those of scientific medicine. Folk medicine combines elements of African culture, European culture, Greek classical medicine, American Indian medicine, scientific medicine, and voodoo religion. These elements are synthesized within the framework of fundamentalist Christianity and provide the participants in the folk medicine system with a broad belief system which allows them to explain illness and misfortunes.

Health, according to this system, is perceived in terms of maintaining a balance between the good and bad forces in the universe. These forces are ever-present, and the individual is continually caught between them; it is generally up to the individual to maintain a harmony between these forces through his or her behavior. Illnesses are classified according to the believed-in causes and are viewed either as natural or unnatural. For example, in a study of root doctors in North Carolina, Quinn and Mathews (n.d.) found that these doctors determine whether an illness is the result of unnatural causes such as spells, in which case it is treated by counter rootwork, or whether it is the result of natural causes and is, therefore, to be treated by herbal or medicinal remedies. Furthermore, root doctors decide whether the illness is predominantly a problem of the body or of the mind. Most illnesses are classified as both (such as nerves and hysterics) and the proper treatment is prescribed accordingly. Indeed, in folk medicine the cause of the illness is more relevant than its symptoms in the diagnosing and treating of illnesses.

Among many Blacks in the South illnesses from natural causes are organized into a belief system based on a theory of balancing the blood in the body. Blood can become unbalanced by being either too sweet ("high blood") or too bitter ("low blood"). Imbalance can be caused from an improper diet (too many sweet or bitter foods), a lack of proper rest, or too much worry. The treatment involves diet modification, family counseling to deal with stressful interpersonal relations and herbal remedies. Furthermore, when blood is not balanced, other bodily fluids may also be out of balance, resulting in an individual's becoming more susceptible to illnesses. Thus, the individual must keep his/her life in balance between the good and evil forces on one hand, and the social and psychological stresses on the other. An imbalance on any of these levels results in illness. At this point, both the popular and scientific medical systems are utilized to restore the balance.

Popular Medicines in Coberly

The people of Coberly use a wide range of medicines other than prescription drugs, including folk medicines and over-the-counter medicines, with 98 percent reporting the use of home remedies. These medicines are used for all their illness episodes, chronic or acute. They are used in addition to "doctor's medicines," generally on a daily or weekly basis, for a variety of ailments including headaches, hypertension, "high blood" and diabetes.

Data were collected on the interview schedule, through in-depth interviewing and through observation of the various remedies used for illnesses. Much of what is reported here is based on what the people of Coberly told me, much of which was validated by the health behavior I observed in their homes and in medical settings over the research period. These data were correlated with the income level and race of respondents (see Table 14); the utilization rates of women and men were also compared. We found that the people of Coberly generally conform to the overall pattern of use of popular medicine in the South.

TABLE 14
Popular Medicine

Illness	Remedy	Type of Remedy/ Preparation	Income of Respondent	Race of Respondent
General pains	Aspirin	Over the counter	$5,000–10,000	B
Diabetes	Insulin Yellow root	Prescription & Over the counter	Less than $5,000	B
Head pain	BC powders	Over the counter	$5,000–10,000	B
Constipation	Feenamint	Over the counter	Less than $5,000	B
Arthritis Stiffness	Liniment	Over the counter	Less than $5,000	B
Rheumatism	Sassafras tea & lemon	Natural plants		B
"Nerves"	Tea & herbs	Natural plants	$5,000–10,000	B
"Nerves"	Yellow root powder	Over the counter	$5,000–10,000	B
Hives	Catnip tea (Catnip plant boiled in water into a tea)	Natural plant	Less than $5,000	B
Upset stomach	Alkaseltzer Cornbread Teas	Over the counter	Less than $5,000	B
Headache	Goody's	Over the counter	$5,000–10,000	B
Constipation	Castor oil	Over the counter	$5,000–10,000	B
Thrash, fever	Yellow root	Over the counter	$5,000–10,000	B
Colds General health problems Menstrual cramps	Yellow root (peel bark off & put in quart of water & tea)	Natural plant	$5,000–10,000	B
Sinus	Antihistamines Sinutab	Over the counter	$10,000– 15,000	B
Chest cold	White whiskey, honey, lemon & vicks (mix to-gether & wrap with cloth around chest & back)	Over the counter	Less than $5,000	B

Illness	Remedy	Type of Remedy/ Preparation	Income of Respondent	Race of Respondent
Wheezing	Elixophyllin, Vitamins, Pheno-barbitol, Iron	Over the counter	$10,000–15,000	B
Cold	Fodder tea	Natural plant		B
Measles	Turpentine (place under bed)	Chemical	Less than $5,000	B
Arthritis	Chlor-Trimeton	Over the counter		B
High blood	Yellow root	Natural plant	Less than $5,000	B
Skin condition	Fresh cow pee & cow manure (cooked & wash person with cow manure)	Animal product	Less than $5,000	B
Heat rash and itch	Poke salad & root tea (apply to skin)	Natural plant	Less than $5,000	B
Fever	Sassafras	Natural plant	Less than $5,000	B
High blood Colds Fever	Pine tea, Garlic Mullein tea (rough leaf)	Natural plants & Herb	Less than $5,000	B
Sinus	Sine-aid	Over the counter	Less than $5,000	B
Colds	Catnip tea Green peachtree leaves Yellow root	Natural plants	$5,000–10,000	B
Stomach problems	Maalox Garlic water	Over the counter & Herb	Less than $5,000	B
Sinus	Honey & water Bufferin	Over the counter & Natural plant	$5,000–10,000	B
Back pain	Ben Gay	Over the counter	$5,000–10,000	B
Thrash	Rabbit tobacco tea with sugar Yellow root with alum water	Natural plants	Less than $5,000	B
Cold	Comtrex	Over the counter	$5,000–10,000	B

(continued)

Illness	Remedy	Type of Remedy/ Preparation	Income of Respondent	Race of Respondent
Cramps	Liniment & water Sticky balls boiled off pinetree	Over the counter & Natural plant	Less than $5,000	B
Chest colds	Mix lard, turpen- tine, Vicks & soda	Natural products & Over the counter	Less than $5,000	B
High blood	Aspirin	Over the counter	Less than $5,000	B
Constipation Colds	Herbs	Natural plants	$5,000–10,000	B
Fever	Green peachtree leaves, cornblade tea (fodder)	Natural plants	Less than $5,000	B
Nerves	Diuretics (from drug store), Nerve pill, Bufferly root	Over the counter & Natural plants	Less than $5,000	B
Colds	Grandmaster Rattlesnake	Natural plants	$5,000–10,000	B
Nerves, burns, ulcers, gastric problems	Goldseal herb with lemon juice	Natural plants	$5,000–10,000	B
Sugar (diabetes) Colds	Rabbit tobacco tea, Poke salad (wash it, juice poison, Dr. suggest cooking)	Natural plant	Less than $5,000	B
Headaches	Tylenol	Over the counter	Less than $5,000	B
Asthma	Rock candy, Whiskey, Pills from drug store	Over the counter & Mineral	Less than $10,000	B
Sores	Sulphur	Mineral	$5,000–10,000	B
Sprain	White vinegar & red mud plaster	Over the counter	$5,000–10,000	B
Flu, Colds	Castor oil	Over the counter	$5,000–10,000	B
Eye problems	Flex seed (smooth like watermelon, v- shaped, black with brown speck)	Natural plant	Less than $5,000	B

Illness	Remedy	Type of Remedy/ Preparation	Income of Respondent	Race of Respondent
Burns	Aloe	Natural pant	$5,000–10,000	B
Body trouble	Flour sack (tie around you while lying down)	Mechanical device	$5,000–10,000	B
Mumps	Marrow of hog jaw & now sardines (rub on mumps)	Animal material	$5,000–10,000	B
Whooping cough	Hoof tea (from hog feet)	Animal material	$5,000–10,000	B
High blood, Fluids, Heart trouble	Inderal & Yellow root	Over the counter & Natural plant	Less than $5,000	B
Sinus	Allerest	Over the counter	$5,000–10,000	B
Diarrhea	Tea from pineburrs	Natural plant	Less than $5,000	B
Indigestion	Metamucil	Over the counter	$15,000–$20,000	W
Tension	Alcohol	Over the counter	$20,000+	W
Cramps	Black pepper tea	Natural herb	$5,000–10,000	W
Headache	Anacin Librium	Over the counter & Prescription	$20,000+	W
Allergies Cold	Sassafras tea Hycomine	Over the counter & Natural plant	$20,000+	W
Constipation	Stool softener Ginseng root tea Black Draught	Over the counter & Natural plant	$20,000+	W
Cold	Lemon tea with whiskey Iron	Over the counter	$20,000+	W
Heart problem	Diuretic (Diozod), Vitamin C, E-B complex	Over the counter	$20,000+	W
Tension	Alcohol	Over the counter	$20,000+	W
Cramps	Hot lemon tea	Natural plant	$5,000–10,000	W

(continued)

Illness	Remedy	Type of Remedy/ Preparation	Income of Respondent	Race of Respondent
Bladder infection	Antibiotic White vinegar & Red mud plaster	Prescription, Over the counter & Natural	$5,000–10,000	W
Headaches	Aspirin	Over the counter	$20,000+	W
Chest cold	Mustard root	Natural plant	$5,000–10,000	W
Cold	Whiskey & sugar, honey, lemon	Over the counter	Less than $5,000	W
Heart palpitation	Inderal, Sassafras tea	Prescription & Natural plant	$20,000+	W
Cold	Castor oil	Over the counter	$15,000–20,000	W
Nerves High blood	Sleeping pills Iron pills Stool softener	Over the counter	$5,000–10,000	W
Constipation Headache	Ginseng root tea Black Draught Tylenol	Natural plant & Over the counter	$10,000–15,000	W
Stings	Snuff or tobacco	Natural plant	$15,000–20,000	W
Heart	Norpacs (100 ml) Diozod (Diuretic)	Prescription & Over the counter	$10,000–15,000	W
Cold, stomach pain, colic	Catnip tea	Natural pant	$5,000–10,000	W
Hives, stomach	Ground ivy	Natural plant	$5,000–10,000	W
Pneumonia	Leaves of tobacco, Moisten with kerosene	Natural plant	$5,000–10,000	W
Foot problems	Tallow w/ Quinine	Over the counter	$10,00–15,000	W
Heart palpitations	Heart leaves (shaped like leaves grown close to ground, wash, dry it & boil)	Natural plant	$10,000–15,000	W
Cold	Pokeberries (Boiled & steam)	Natural plant	$5,000–10,000	W

Illness	Remedy	Type of Remedy/ Preparation	Income of Respondent	Race of Respondent
Side pleurisy, low blood	Poke root, new onion, Bufferin (wash, cut up and boil root, make poultice while it is warm, stir in corn meal)	Natural plant & Over the counter	$5,000–10,000	W
Indigestion	Baking soda with aspirin, Gout pills	Over the counter	$5,000–10,000	W
Headache	Alkaseltzer Estrogen Librium	Prescription & Over the counter	$20,000+	W
Asthma	Rock candy & Whiskey	Over the counter	$5,000–10,000	W
Sprain	Mustard & leaves from pine tree	Natural plant	$5,000–10,000	W
Cold	Cough syrup Sassafras tea	Over the counter & Natural plant	$5,000–10,000	W
Cold	Lemon, honey & whiskey	Over the counter	Less than $5,000	W
Laxative	Black Draught	Over the counter	$5,000–10,000	W
Cold	Horehound leaves	Natural plant	Less than $5,000	W
Bad feeling in upper chest Constipation	Epsom salts	Over the counter	Less than $5,000	W
Shortness of breath—prevent heart attack	Nitrol ointment	Over the counter	$5,000–10,000	W
Arthritis	Mullet tea	Natural plant	Less than $5,000	W
Stomach ache	Tums	Over the counter	Less than $15,000	W
Earache	Drop of beetle blood	Animal product	Less than $15,000	W
Constipation	Feenamint	Over the counter	$10,000–15,000	W

More women than men use traditional rather than medically prescribed medicines, and Blacks use them more than Whites. White females use more over-the-counter medicines and only a few "folk medicines"—they use mostly aspirin or other pain-killers, vitamins, and pills for a variety of ailments, as well as teas and other folk remedies. Black women use by far the widest range of natural and over-the-counter medicines. They trust them for certain health problems more than a doctor's medicines. Their reasons for using home remedies are: (1) they are familiar with the products because they see them advertised on television ("media medicine"), and (2) they are familiar with the popular medicines because they have been transmitted from generation to generation and are thus a part of their cultural model for preventive and curative health care.

Black women and men discussed the medicines they would use in the past when "there was no doctor" (meaning they lacked access to one). They also talked about what would happen when their relatives and friends were ill in the past. Usually an older woman would "doctor" them with the best medicines she knew. Sometimes a physician would come. More often, however, the ill person would get well with the use of a "healer" and traditional medicines. Some said they did not use these alternatives anymore because they are "no longer available"; "it is difficult to obtain the roots and herbs to make teas anymore." Women in the past would harvest herbs every year and either sell them or give them to people to use in preparing remedies. Only a few of these women are still active in healing, and these are still giving advice about the use of certain roots for specific illnesses. People also once obtained roots from the "raleighman" who kept jars of medicine (herbs). Evidently, these men no longer exist in Coberly. They are currently found in nearby urban areas, where they are known as "root doctors," herbalists or nutritional specialists. Some Coberlians travel to the city to see these specialists or send someone there to get "medicines." Often they "know someone" who will bring the medicines to Coberly.

White women use over-the-counter drugs more often than Black women do, and the older white women have switched to "drug store medicines" or "doctor's medicines" from the use of "teas" in recent years. Whites have a longer tradition of being able to afford "doctor's medicines" and over-the-counter medicines. Therefore, compared to Blacks, Whites have linked into the biomedical cultural model for a longer period of time and have more linkages to "medicines" that cost money. Blacks have linked more into traditional medicines and healers and have only recently incorporated a large quantity of over-the-counter medicines and medical resources in general (again, a problem of access). This accounts for the slight difference in health beliefs between poor Blacks and Whites, and reflects the connection between health behavior and beliefs.

Knowledge of popular medicines reported in Coberly is generally trans-mitted from mother to daughter, although men who have special knowledge of healing will transmit the knowledge to women. The "medicines" are used for a variety of health problems, including colds, headaches, arthritis, diabetes, back pain, rash, constipation, high blood, low blood, and "nerves." The use of laxatives is common and is related to the general belief that one's body becomes polluted from overeating or from taking too much medicine. Overeating occurs generally at social occassions such as Christmas, Thanksgiving and birthdays and at recurrent gatherings such as homecomings and campmeetings; the remedy is taking a laxative to rid the body of impurities.

Because their access to medical facilities has been fairly recent, it is not surprising that lower income people use more popular medicines than upper income people in Coberly. A majority of upper income people said that they do not believe in such medicines and exhibited a hostile attitude toward them. They did, paradoxically, report using chiropractors, taking vitamins, drinking alcoholic beverages and taking prescription medicines such as Valium for their health. The media and Medicare, moreover, have had a leveling effect on the use of prescription and over-the-counter medicines. All income levels now use them. Consequently, the differential behavior now seems to be the use of "holistic modalities" by middle and upper income people and the use of "folk medicines" by lower income people. Both can be categorized, no matter what they're called, as popular medicine.

Community studies conducted in rural areas several years ago found similar cultural models of popular medicine and health. In a small rural town of 300 in the Missouri Ozarks, Withers (1946) found that the older people believed in witches and diviners and that most of the people used home remedies for symptomatic treatment of self-diagnosed ailments—what he called "a kind of pseudorational practice associated with orthodox medical practice involving extensive use of patent medicines." Knowledge about the use and preparation of the home remedies was very widespread. Likewise, Koos (1954) reported the use of home remedies in Regionville, a community in upstate New York. Yet, definitions of illness, beliefs about causation, attitudes toward medical care and medical practitioners and responses to illness were strongly related to social class—findings similar to those reported for Coberly.

Use of Traditional Healers in Coberly

Use of traditional healers by the people of Coberly is directly related to their knowledge and beliefs concerning the effectiveness of specialists other than medical personnel. The persistence of belief in and use of popular specialists is a function of the cultural and economic system in this society. Although upper income Whites use alternative healers such as chiropractors and naturopaths, they are either unaware of or do not utilize the informal traditional healers in the community as do lower income Whites and Blacks. Nonetheless, about half the people of Coberly said they use some kind of healer other than medical doctors. Lower income Whites consult a specialist such as an herbalist or a healer for conjuring warts, curing the thrash (thrush) and talking the fire out of burns. All of the older people had used such healers and had taken their children. The younger people (under 40) said that their parents or grandparents had taken them to such healers when they were young, but that they now utilize a medical doctor except for sometimes consulting the "thrashman" about their children.

Coberly Blacks are very knowledgeable about folk specialists and the older ones (above 40) talked at length about their use of and belief in the popular specialists. Like poor Whites, Blacks used these healers more in the past than they do now. Many of the healers they discussed are old or have died in the past few years. Cultural models that include knowledge of the variety of healers used in the past are not being transmitted to the younger generation. Only information about root doctors, thrash men or women and the use of teas and herbs are still very much in the health cultural system. The use of midwives, healers who "stop blood," and "fire talkers" has subsided in recent years.

The people who do use these healers feel that they can help people with certain problems "better than a doctor." Some see healers for all their problems in addition to seeing doctors. One woman saw a healer when she had "female problems"—she said "when the body falls." The doctor told her to sit in a tub of epsom salts which, according to her, didn't help. Then her mother told her to swing from doors, which also didn't help. Her mother then took her to "a woman who could help" who inserted a flour sack which had been soaked in a solution of vaseline, turpentine and salt. This sack had a string attached and was inserted like a tampon. When the sack was pulled out, her "body came back up and she was cured."

Another person saw a woman who made a solution of fatback and castor oil and rubbed it in the mouth of her baby with a white rag. This healer is believed to have a lot of power. She goes to the houses of both Blacks and Whites who are ill and prays for them. Indeed, as other studies have reported, black and white clients utilize healers of either ethnic group. The reputation of the healer and his/her ability to heal overrides the ethnic factor in choosing a folk healer.

Blacks talked about conditions under which they lived in the past and how they could not see a doctor or use the clinical facilities and hospitals. They "had to take care of themselves with home remedies or go to someone who knew remedies or knew how to heal." They are aware and thankful that they now have access to scientific medicine and, as we have seen, they utilize it with frequency. Scientific medicine is now a part of their health cultural model. It also includes popular medicine, as does that of Whites. Elsewhere, I have analyzed the traditional folk medical system in the rural South (Hill 1973, 1976, 1981) and concluded that it is (1) an adaptation to the economic position of poor people in the social structure, (2) a system of beliefs and behaviors that provides an explanation for illnesses and healings and allows people to cope, both physically and mentally, with either their lack of access to the health care system, or their treatment (physically and behaviorally) in the health care system, and (3) a part of a broad integrated system of beliefs and behavior that also incorporates their knowledge of the scientific medical system.

Causal Explanations for Illness and Healing

Causal explanations are a crucial part of understanding a belief system. The people of Coberly have beliefs that not only guide and reflect their behavioral patterns but also provide explanations for why people become ill, the kinds of people who are more likely to become ill, their choices of health alternatives, their compliance behavior, their health prevention behavior, their explanation for getting well and their place in the health structure. Coberlians' patterns of explanation vary according to ethnicity and income levels, with Blacks believing in a wider array of causal factors and lower income Blacks and Whites expressing similar beliefs, while upper income Whites believe in what they think is the scientific model and following that model, place more reliance on natural causes of diseases. Not surprising, the heterogeneity of the community is reflected in their cultural models, as in their behavior.

For Whites, the major causes of illness are natural causes, social causes and emotional causes. The natural causes are mostly biological and include agents such as germs, viruses, heredity, the effects of weather and malfunctions in the body. This category was primarily used by upper income Whites to explain their illnesses and refers to acute, severe, chronic, and temporary illnesses. Typical examples of the responses of Coberly Whites when asked what sorts of things cause illness are: "acting bad," "partly heredity, partly social contact," "not taking care of oneself," "lack of good eating habits and exercise," "overeating," "physical and mental factors," and "germs, viruses and stress."

Social or behavioral causes are most frequently cited by Whites as causes for most illnesses. Within this category most frequently mentioned are inappropriate eating behavior (such as overeating or not eating the right foods), lack of exercise, or not wearing the proper clothes during winter. In addition, these Coberlians believe that contact with sick people and breaking the community norms can cause illness. Nearly all of these explanations are aimed at individual behavior, a fact which reflects a strong belief in individual responsibility and explains the frequently discussed explanation of "self" as a causal agent. Our interviewees stated that drinking and eating too much and just not taking care of oneself cause illness more often than do natural causes. Upper income Whites combined these causes with germs and other natural causes such as heredity.

Furthermore, many Whites relate social causes to emotional or psychological ones. The third most frequently cited cause was "stress" or "mental difficulty," the latter often related to individual behavior. The statement "Your mind can cause illness" reflects a belief that one's state of mind is important for good or bad health. Overeating, for example, is deemed a mental or emotional problem of the individual which will cause illness. A small percentage of Whites, mostly upper income ones, related overwork to stress and felt that if the pressure becomes too great, illness results. Overall, Whites integrate these categories through relating them to specific behaviors that are, more often than not, controllable by the individual. A majority of Whites in Coberly believe that specific kinds of people are sick more often than others. They feel that certain people complain about illnesses to get attention and even go to doctors more often for attention. These people are generally older or people who want attention because they need love. One person commented, "they're ignored so they do whatever will get some attention when they need it. Everyone needs love." In addition, people who are jealous of others' getting attention will themselves complain about illnesses. Other kinds of people who suffer from illness more often than others are older people, inactive people, children and "abused kids," people under stress who worry a lot, lonely people, people with "weak constitutions," those who are "more susceptible to germs," people who can't or don't eat properly, people with dangerous jobs, women (female problems), and victims of heredity.

Whites have a different permutation of variables than Blacks that provide them with causal explanations for illnesses. Sometimes they couched their explanations in moral terms. Although they seldom invoked explicitly religious teachings, their comments about smokers, poor nutrition, and misplaced values (physical, moral and mental behavior) were framed in moral terms. The phrase "the people who don't take care of themselves" was rarely used, but the phrases "irresponsible people" and "individual responsibility," were dispersed throughout their dialogues. Whites of Coberly feel strongly that people who do not take responsibility for their health, as reflected in their health behavior, are more likely to become ill. Only about 10 percent of the Whites framed their answers in overtly religious terms. However, when asked if they pray for people who are ill, 45 percent responded that they do, although they qualified their answers with "if it is severe" or "it can't hurt." On the other hand, 95 percent of Blacks said they pray for ill people, and their feeling toward prayer was expressed more strongly. They said, for example, "it is very important," "that is the key for everyone getting well," or "healing and knowledge come from the Lord."

The Blacks of Coberly believe in natural environmental causes of illnesses, social causes and supernatural causes, again integrated, but seen as levels of explanation depending on the specific illness. Supernatural and social causes were discussed most often. God, as a punishing spirit, is believed to be the major reason why people get sick. As one person said, "if people do right, they do better about sickness." Only one person said that the devil is a causal agent. Sinful behavior such as drinking, smoking or eating too much is a reflection of a lack of belief in the Lord. "Not living right," then, is empirical evidence that a person does not believe enough in God, and is consequently breaking a moral code in the community.

These supernatural causes obviously integrate with social causes, which Blacks, like Whites, reduce to individual behavior. Diet is, by far, the most commonly cited cause of illness. Indeed, food is a symbol of health, and the kind and amount one eats represent to the Blacks and poor Whites of Coberly the overall status, including health status, of one's family. Just having enough food to eat is a constant concern. Not only do these groups have to worry about having the money to purchase food in general, they also worry, partly because of recent emphasis by medical personnel, and the media, about purchasing what they have learned is the "right kind of food," or "food that is good for you."

Blacks believe that for the most part the individual is in control of his/her health and illnesses. The social causes of illness discussed by Blacks are, in many ways, similar to those specified by Whites. Individual behavior that leads to illness is, however, always placed by Blacks within the context of religious teachings. As stated above, the most frequently invoked cause of illness is "bad diet," with the second most frequently reported cause in this category being "not acting right," a phrase that refers to both supernatural and natural causes. Social causes are linked to both chronic and acute illnesses.

A small percentage of Blacks (about 10 percent), unlike Whites, expressed a rather fatalistic attitude about illness. The statements "It is just going to happen," or "it's just nature," are typical metaphors expressing a general feeling of lack of control over one's own destiny. These people feel that outside forces such as weather, pollution, drugs, old age or just life are causing them to get sick and that basically no one can do anything to prevent illnesses. Germs are discussed infrequently by Blacks.

Blacks believe that people get well only with the help of the Lord. Ultimately, they feel, it is up to God's will whether someone recovers from illness. Factors like social and individual responsibility are also important to them and integrate into different levels in their explanation of healing. If illness occurs because of behaviors, then logically it can be healed by changing those behaviors. And, indeed, this is the logic of black Coberlians. When one gets sick because of poor diet, then obviously the ill person should change his/her diet. Thus, ideally, Blacks should refrain from eating certain kinds of foods, like pork, and buy more nutritious foods. At this point, however, the interrelationship between beliefs and behavior breaks down. Blacks, like poor Whites, do not have the money to purchase different foods, or they may be unaware of the foods they should purchase, a topic previously discussed.

Inextricably bound to the behavioral aspects of healing, the "power of the mind" and self-responsibility in healing were discussed by Blacks. Phrases such as "the mind has a lot to do with getting well," "everyone can help themselves," and "you have to help yourself," were typically followed by examples of people hurt or dying because they didn't believe in themselves or the Lord. So the mental and moral attitudes of ill people are crucial to their recovery. Not only do they have to care about getting well, but others must care as well, either friends or family. As stated earlier, Blacks do not believe that the doctor heals them as much as Whites believe this. Doctors and their medicine can help, but so do the family, special healers, home remedies and God. These alternative causal agents and behaviors are not in the least mutually exclusive in the minds and behaviors of the black people of Coberly.

Whites in Coberly, on the other hand, refer to supernatural healing much less frequently, and most references are from lower income groups. So the power of God to heal is a causal agent for Whites to a limited degree. To lower income groups, God may be the ultimate healer, but to higher income groups the ultimate factor in healing is the mind. As stated in a previous section, Whites also believe that the doctor and his medicines are the most effective forces for healing. To understand these beliefs, they must be placed in a wider context, one that integrates mind and body in a system similar to that of the Blacks, although varying in content. "The mind" means an attitude and self-concept associated with health behaviors. For example, when a person eats foods that are deemed "not good for him," then this attitude toward food, located in the mind, is controlling the person and he must take responsibility for the behavior. The mind is also closely associated with the "self" in that the self can control the mind. So we have a feedback loop between the mind, which can heal, and the self which takes responsibility for the behavior. As one person said, "one's attitude (mind) determines behavior and response to illness." Other typical phrases used about the healing process were, "it is important to believe in yourself," "you have to want to get better," "the body heals itself," "personal discipline and taking responsibility for oneself" and "the body heals itself, mind over matter."

Another causal agent separate from the mind/self, albeit cognitively and behaviorally related, is the physical level, i.e., the level of scientific medicine. People become ill because of germs or heredity, so most commonly seek help from the medical profession. And it is up to the person to comply with the treatment. Again, upper income people comply more often and seek medical treatment more quickly and frequently than lower income Whites. White Coberlians in general, however, believe that people should follow the doctor's prescribed treatments; it is a part of their responsibility for the self. Taking medicine is believed to be similar to eating properly or exercising. Some people said that if one has a positive attitude it not only makes one feel better but also makes medicine work faster. Thus, complying with doctor's orders is just one part of the healing process, the other part being the beliefs and attitudes of a person.

While all people of Coberly feel that there is a uniformity in causes of illness and everyone has an equal chance of becoming ill, the majority believe that there are specific kinds of people who become ill more than others. People can get sick because of their behavior and they can also get well because of their behavior (i.e., relationship to family, community, environment and God). Black causal beliefs incorporate: (1) physical behavior, i.e., poor diet due to "inadequate food" or inactivity, and (2) moral/mental behavior such as "worrying too much," or "not living right." Both of these categories, in the minds of Coberly's Blacks, incorporate taking responsibility for oneself. In fact, the phrase "people get sick because they do not take care of themselves," was recorded over and over in the interviews. Another prevelant belief among Blacks is that people who "do not live the way the Lord wants them to will get sick more often." Again, this refers not only to "eating and sleeping right," but to "living right," i.e., living according to the teachings of God and living up to His moral standards. Indeed, all the behaviors that Blacks believe will cause illnesses are framed within their ideas about the moral order.

White causal beliefs also emphasize the importance of the individual in causing his/her illnesses. They rely less on supernatural causes and more on natural causes such as germs and stress. But, as discussed above, the beliefs of lower income Whites are more similar to those of Blacks than to those of upper income Whites. This group talked more about the moral order and God, indicating a closer integration of natural and supernatural causes. The few upper income Whites have separated this cause-and-effect link and use the cultural model set out by scientific medicine.

Whites and Blacks, then, have a broad framework that includes more than scientific medicine's knowledge concerning illness and healing, although both incorporate (at different levels) the scientific model. Both groups also feel that their beliefs and behaviors are a part of the healing process. One person expressed this by stating, "We want to be active along with the doctor in getting well." Whether all the people of Coberly are consciously aware of this belief, they certainly expressed it in their statements and reflected it in their verbal behaviors. They believe that a person's state of mind is important for healing. This sense of "partnership" with the significant others in the illness and healing process is clearer when their health beliefs are analyzed within the context of their health behaviors.

Cultural Models of the Medical System

The people of Coberly respond behaviorially in various ways to their illnesses and the initiation of health-seeking behaviors (Chapters 3 and 4). They act, and they react to the information they seek out or are given concerning health and illnesses. Their actions, as we have seen, vary according to ethnic background and income level, two important variables that determine the kind of information people are exposed to. Behavior is also guided by the cultural models people build up, which are elaborated on as new information is incorporated, and this new information is perceived as consistent with their perceived social and physical lives. In this way, Coberlians are able to incorporate the scientific model of health into their traditional belief system without a sense of conflict. People thus expand their models as new information is obtained and, as we have seen, these models are heterogeneous for the small community of Coberly. Exhibiting the behaviors described in Chapters 3 and 4, then, makes perfect sense to them.

Beliefs and the cultural models built up from them are the basis for understanding how people link to the medical system. People's ideas about the causes and effects of illness and health are important, as we saw in the last section. Relating them to the behavior previously described allows us to explain why people's behavior appears to be in conflict with the expectations of medical personnel. In this section, I will discuss Coberlians' beliefs about medical doctors, their compliance with medical treatment, and the financing of medical care.

The Key Mediator: The Medical Doctor

Two key links between people and the medical system are doctors and nurses. The often-quoted phrase in this society "the doctor is a God," and the reverential treatment of doctors, do not hold true for the people of Coberly. If one word would describe most of their beliefs about doctors it is "questioning." All income and ethnic groups believe the doctor "knows best" sometimes. Although a few patterns emerged that differentiated Blacks and Whites, the majority of both groups extensively discussed why they believe the doctor either knows or does not know about illness. About 70 percent felt that doctors can help one get well; 12 percent said doctors could not help and the remainder said they sometimes help one get well. A smaller percentage (66 percent) think the doctor sometimes knows best about one's health. Only 12 percent said they believe the doctor never knows best about their health. In our discussions, Coberlians delineated the categories of illness episodes for which they believe doctors can and cannot be effective in their treatments, and discussed how the medical behavior of doctors has affected their lives both positively and negatively.

The types of illnesses doctors are more effective in treating are ones which people themselves cannot diagnose: those with unfamiliar symptoms or those that people have had little or no experience with. In these cases they go to the doctor with a "fuzzy" diagnosis. Many people, both Blacks and Whites, believe that the doctor knows best about illnesses that he/she can use equipment and tests to diagnose. These cases involve the knowledge and utilization of machines that go beyond the illness experience of the people in measuring bodily functions and malfunctions. Such knowledge, gained in medical school, makes doctors, in the minds of the people of Coberly, effective in treating illnesses such as kidney and liver malfunctions, those requiring surgery, and those that need to be monitored by machines.

Religious preference and ethnic background appear to be significant factors in choosing and utilizing a doctor. Although most of the people of Coberly (93 percent) said they would go to a female doctor, only 36 percent would see a "foreign doctor." Over 65 percent think that doctors should believe in God; this is clearly an important factor in choosing a doctor. While over 42 percent (black and white) said they would not use a black doctor, the majority think that they might, "if he is a good one."

Believing that doctors are fallible and make mistakes, most people of Coberly change doctors if they feel one is not helping them. Since all doctors cannot always be right, another may be better and the only way to find out is to "get another opinion" or "shop around." These reponses came from more of the lower income people, whereas higher income respondents tend to stay with their family doctors and infrequently change doctors. They have routinely utilized doctors' services for a longer period of time and have the tradition of a family doctor. According to the medical personnel in the county, changing doctors is a major problem. It is difficult, they say, to keep up with individual records and treatment patterns, a problem which they think lowers the quality of health care.

White Coberlians emphasize the training, education and diagnostic abilities of doctors, and talked about their experiences with doctors which led them to question the doctors' effectiveness. One person said, "they are wrong sometimes; they misdiagnosed my daughter several times so I went to another town." Another person wonders "why doctors have to ask us what is wrong and I don't understand why they can't just examine us and tell us what is wrong." Still another black man said, "When I have tried everything else, I then go to a doctor. When I do go, I do what he says." A black woman responded to us by saying, "doctors do not know best all the time. You know more than they do about what's hurting. They also sometimes give the wrong medications." One white man stated, "doctors are like automobile mechanics, they will always find something wrong." Another said, "doctors are human and aren't perfect. They don't know everything. Younger doctors are better than older ones since older doctors have hard-to-change habits." Yet several people remembered the family doctor of years ago who knew everything that was wrong with the family members. Indeed, several said "the younger doctors ignore the patient's information, and they don't know how you really feel; they don't have your feelings." These discrepancies in expected use of medical personnel are based on different cultural models of health behavior which are inextricably bound to peoples' beliefs about doctors and their beliefs about their own control over their health and health behavior.

When questioned further about their beliefs concerning the reasons doctors help people get well, a larger percentage of Whites than Blacks stated they believe that the doctor, because of his training and education, can help one's illness: "They know what to look for, they went to school." A majority discussed training and knowledge of technology and science as the key reasons for doctors' abilities in the health field. They delineated specific situations in which a doctor is most effective—all related to his/her diagnostic capabilities, use of antibiotics and ability to stop pain through prescribed drugs. Several added, however, that such help is only temporary and they will have to continue to visit the doctor and pay more money. Indeed, many Whites feel that doctors just want to make money. About 10 percent believe that the doctor heals through the Lord, while an equal number told us that "doctors only experiment with people; they do not care." One person said that the reason doctors heal (if they do) is due to the caring they have for their patients.

The Blacks of Coberly reported a wider range of reasons why the doctor can help a person with "illnesses" than Whites. Probing on this question revealed once again the belief in the individual's ability to heal him/herself. Over 30 percent said that the "self," not the doctor, ultimately heals itself. Another fifth of the Black respondents said that they heal only with the Lord's help. Typical answers were "sometimes they (doctors) don't do any good; the ones who get well are the ones the Lord wants to"; "they try, a lot depends on helping yourself and God"; "doctors administer medicines but God heals"; "people get well because they have hope and faith they're gonna get well"; and lastly, "you get yourself well with a good attitude or if a person wants to." These are the reasons why the doctor does not and cannot help people get well. Additional reasons why doctors do not help are "they don't talk enough," "they choose the people they want to help," and "they are too specialized." Like Whites, the Blacks of Coberly feel that doctors can only heal certain types of illnesses such as "very serious problems," "only physical problems," or diabetes and heart problems, the major health problems for which they seek medical help.

In contrast to previous analyses of the poor in rural Southern settings, I found that the people of Coberly have a general feeling of control rather than an attitude of fatalism about their health. Such beliefs permeate all their answers concerning beliefs and attitudes. These outlooks are reflected in their own words such as (1) "I know myself best"; (2) "If I know what's wrong, I can go and do something for myself just as well"; (3) "I have to take care of myself and not rely on doctors"; (4) "Each individual knows their own body better"; (5) "People can tell the doctor what's wrong with them more often"; and (6) "I would not turn my life over to them and say do what you want with me." These statements are representative of the general beliefs and attitudes toward doctors and their medicine. The people of Coberly feel that they can make judgements about their own health, including utilization of health resources and compliance with the doctor's treatment.

Compliance with Medical Treatment

One of the major health problems reported by medical personnel in Coberly is that of compliance by the people with prescribed treatments. When Coberlians seek medical help for a health problem, they often do not comply with the doctor's treatment orders and they are aware that they do not, even though they have linked with the medical system. Compliance with prescribed medical treatment is directly related to their beliefs about what can help a person get well. As described in a previous section, the people of Coberly often question the effectiveness of medical advice and told us about illness episodes in which they did not comply or only partially complied with the doctor's advice. All Coberlians discussed times when they decided not to follow the doctor's instructions. By far, however, the group that most frequently does not comply is Blacks; they questioned "doctor's medicine" more often, whereas Whites more often discussed their "trust" in the doctor's advice. Many people said they did not comply with the doctor's instructions because they feel that, at times, they know best how to treat themselves. Non-compliance, a behavior that demonstrates a sense of confidence in one's own knowledge and individual responsibility and thus control of the doctor/patient relationship, was encountered among all Coberlians, but less so among middle- and upper income people.

Coberlians' stated reasons for compliance or non-compliance are varied and reflect their general perception of a doctor and his/her ability to heal, and the level of their trust in a healer. Whites follow doctors' instructions for such reasons as, "Why else go to him"; "they are educated and dedicated and know what they are doing"; and, more frequently, "trust." Most Whites follow doctors' instructions, the reason being that they trust him/her. A majority said "what else can I do," indicating that they do not have very many options in their illness behavior model. Some feel that the doctor is the last resort and when the decision to visit him is made, it is the individual's responsibility to comply with the prescribed treatment. Others "sometimes" comply because (1) they use home remedies that help more, (2) the side-effects of medicines are unpleasant, or (3) they cannot afford all the medicines. Several people showed me the Valium a doctor had prescribed for "nerves" or bursitus. One black woman took one and threw the others away saying, "It didn't help and made me crazy." Others said that they did not take the number of pills they were supposed to everyday. Other reasons for non-compliance were "instructions are too rough," "sometimes use home remedies instead; they work better" or "if side effects are unpleasant or dangerous." No one discussed outright refusing to comply with doctors' prescribed treatments.

In contrast to Whites, about 20 percent of the Blacks of Coberly reported that they usually do not do what the doctor tells them to. Their reasoning is that doctors "are just pill pushers," that the treatment "often does not work"; "I know better"; or "it makes me feel worse." A majority of Blacks "sometimes" comply depending on whether they judge the medicine helpful. They discussed situations in which they would comply such as severe pain and other acute episodes but hastily added that when they felt better, they would stop taking the medicine. Many persons reported cases in which the doctor prescribed medicines for ailments that they did not have or medicines that did not work. For example, they said the doctor "told me to take these pills for a headache, but I did not have a headache so I did not take them."

Several said they would comply "if I feel it is right for me" or "when I think it will help." A majority feel that if they go to a doctor they should attempt to follow the treatment, i.e., if they had made the effort to consult a doctor, his advice should be considered. As one person said "there is no sense in going if you don't try to follow instructions." Only a few Blacks discussed trust as an important reason for complying with a doctor's orders. The Blacks who "sometimes" comply with medical treatment generally think that they can judge whether the medicines help them. One person stated that she complied, "only when I feel it is right for me and if it is not, I stop taking the medicine." Another man said, "I take doctor's medicines only when I think they help," while another stated, "the person knows best about taking medicines so I take it only when I feel it is necessary."

Blacks who comply most of the time do so for a variety of reasons. Unlike Whites, only a small number feel that trust is the key reason, while a larger number go to a doctor only when they have a serious problem and "when I go, I do what they say." Blacks respect doctors and feel they know what is best under certain circumstances. Contrary to most Whites, they do not trust a doctor completely with their health fate. They take more of an active role in the treatment of their health problems.

More women than men use home remedies in conjunction with prescribed medicines, and more women say that they comply completely with doctors' orders. Even though men seek help from doctors less frequently than women, when they do so, most feel that they should attempt to comply with their prescriptions. Furthermore, the higher their income, the more trust people have in doctors and the higher their degree of compliance. The highest income group, for example, said they complied because doctors are "educated and dedicated" and that they felt that the doctor knows best. As we descend the income levels, and ascend in age, compliance is less common and is more frequently combined with home remedies.

Several examples of types of compliance behavior were discussed in Chapters 3 and 4. These usually involve illnesses for which people also take popular medicines, and they think that taking the medicine from the doctor and supplementing it with natural and/or over-the-counter medicines would be taking "too much medicine." So, they make decisions about how much of each would bring about the proper balance and make them well. Other reasons for not complying at all are the negative side-effects of certain medicines and the trouble taking medicines, changing diet or exercising causes in their lives. Compliance behavior clearly demonstrates the correlation between people's cultural models and their behavior, which often is considered a problem by the medical personnel in Coberly.

The Case of Mr. and Mrs. Taylor

Mr. and Mrs. Taylor are a white couple in their seventies. They live by themselves and have no relatives in Coberly, but a son lives 20 miles away and visits on Sundays. Mr. Taylor worked for 45 years as a farmer. He owned a little piece of land that produced cotton in the early days and later soybeans, a few peanuts and corn. As he said, "I never had much but I made a living and had enough to raise a family." Mrs. Taylor has always been a housewife. They met at a local dance in Coberly and married six months later. Having lived all their lives in Coberly, they generally feel that "things have changed for the worse, people used to be nicer and the young people were good." Both have been diagnosed as having high blood pressure and Mrs. Taylor has diabetes. They use Medicaid and "make a trip to the doctor about once a month." Everytime they go the doctor prescribes a medicine for their 'high blood,' and before going home they have the prescription filled at the pharmacy. On the dresser in their bedrooms, they have over 30 bottles of the medicine lined up in order of the dates they purchased them. They asked me several times if I thought the doctor was giving them the right medicines. Mr. Taylor said that he did not trust the doctor when the cure was worse than the problem. He thinks this is particularly true when it comes to cancer—"all those radiation treatments that make you sick." The side-effects of the hypertensive medicine make them "feel crazy," sometimes dizzy and faint. Because of this, they take it infrequently; maybe two or three times a week at most. Everyday, however, they drink a tea made from yellow root twice a day, which they believe "helps high blood as much as other medicines." They frequently discussed the doctor's orders concerning their diet. "He wants us to stop eating what we have eaten all our lives"; and "on top of that, the things he wants us to eat cost more money." They showed me their checks from "the welfare office" and said they cannot afford to do what the doctor says. "Anyway, all those things don't taste good so why should I change now?" Mrs. Taylor had similar comments about her compliance with the doctor's orders to treat her diabetes. Again, she does not take all the medicine he gives her since yellow root controls diabetes as well as "high blood." Since her case is not severe, she pays little attention to his orders although they purchase all the medicine he prescribes. They have no intention of changing their eating habits and believe that "other things" can be good treatments besides the things prescribed by the doctor. The "certain circumstances" under which the Taylors are more amenable to strictly following the doctor's orders are those that manifest severe pain or a potential disability or a clear vision of impending death. Mrs. Taylor had an operation several years ago for a hernia. It caused her so much pain that she was willing to do anything the doctor said to stop it. A further reason for compliance was that "he was going to cut on me—I could have died." It is clear that Mr. and Mrs. Taylor activate their cultural model of cause-and-effect and decide what and how much medicines are good for them.

The Case of Helen

Helen is a 28-year-old black woman who is head of a household consisting of her 14-year-old daughter, two sons (ages 12 and 10) and her nine-month-old daughter. She had been pregnant with another child that died just after delivery. Helen works at a local factory as a secretary. She learned to type in high school and took a six-week course at a nearby junior college. At that time, her mother was living and helped take care of the children she had as an adolescent. Helen first became pregnant at the age of 14 because she "didn't know what she was doing." All she wanted at the time was attention from a man, to feel like a woman and to do what she said was, she thought, a way of keeping him. She knew that her mother would take care of her and her child so she could finish school. By the time she was in the eleventh grade, she had two children and decided to drop out and work. When she first became pregnant (she knew because she "missed two months"), she told her mother and grandmother. They were supportive and helped her as much as they could through the pregnancy (and the other three). They gave her teas to drink regularly and would recommend "over-the-counter" medicines for any problems she encountered. She went to the public health clinic once to see what they had to say about pregnancy but was "lectured" by the nurse, so she decided not to go again. "Anyway, Mama knows more and all they talked about was eating habits. Not to eat this and that and not to gain weight. I believe that doesn't matter. God gave me the baby and He wants it to be healthy, not starved to death. My family knows best."

Not only did Helen not comply with the advice of the public health nurse about her first child, she didn't comply with her advice about the second either. She delivered the first child at home with a midwife attending to the birth; her family did not have enough money to pay a doctor or the hospital. For the third and fourth child, they saved the money and borrowed some from relatives. Toward the end of each of these pregnancies, Helen went to see the doctor who would deliver her babies. Her experience with the second child became one of those "certain circumstances" in which she thought that "the doctor knows best." She had some trouble with the pregnancy, so she consulted a doctor in the eighth month; he told her she might lose the baby. At that point, she complied with his prescriptions and "tried to do what he said." She took the medicines along with the teas and herbs given her by her grandmother. She also prayed to God and began to "look to Him for guidance." Today, she thinks that God helped her much more than the doctor, who only cost her money. In fact, it was always difficult to find doctors who would deliver the baby(ies); Helen had to prove to them that she had the money to pay before they would consent to have her admitted into the hospital to deliver a baby. The second baby was born but died three days later. So, during the subsequent two pregnancies, she consulted a doctor earlier. She still did not comply with all the dieting advice or take all the medicines he prescribed, however, and "they came out all right." The doctor gave her pills to take after every meal. She is still confused about how often he meant. She eats only two meals a day and wonders if he meant three times a day.

Another "certain circumstance" in Helen's life in which she participated in complying with the prescription of the medical system was when her mother had cancer. "We knew something was wrong long before the doctor found out what it was—she was losing weight and feeling real bad all the time. The teas didn't do any good or the medicines the man up there in Magnolia told her to take. We knew that she needed those tests the doctor gives in his office and finally they told [the doctor] what was wrong. She had cancer in her lower intestines. She was operated on and when she came home, she recovered enough to get around the house. At first, she had to go for those Cobalt treatments that made her sick. She didn't want to go, but I made her. I thought they would help. She took most of the medicine the doctor gave her and drank special teas everyday. She really thought that only God could save her." Two years after her operation Helen's mother became severely ill and died. Helen thinks that the doctors did all they could, they just didn't know enough to save her. Like most people in Coberly, Helen makes her own decisions about how and when and from whom to seek health care and the degree to which she complies with their treatments.

Compliance with the prescriptions of the medical system involves a complex of behaviors and beliefs which illustrate the cultural models of the people of Coberly. Such models are different for different subpopulations, but, as we have seen in previous chapters, all people expand the medical cultural model as they respond to illness. Compliance is a matter of degree; it depends upon the individual's cultural, social, and economic circumstances. Variability in compliance, therefore, is not surprising among and within the ethnic and income groups that make up the social structure of Coberly.

The Financing of Medical Care

Like those about compliance or preventive health, beliefs and attitudes about the financing of medical care guide people's linkages to the medical system. We asked people what they thought about government subsidies for health services to the poor and elderly and how their ideas affected their own health behavior. As with other aspects of their behavior, the cultural models of the people of Coberly vary according to ethnicity and income level. Blacks and lower income Whites share similar beliefs regarding the reasons Medicare and Medicaid should continue to exist. All Blacks in Coberly believe they are poor and indeed, they do represent the lower end of the income levels in the community. Most receive aid from the government for health care, as do most of the lower income Whites. Not surprisingly, their beliefs and values are quite different from those of upper income Whites, most of whom do not receive financial aid and have rather negative attitudes toward Medicare/Medicaid.

Blacks overwhelmingly believe that the poor are not responsible for being poor. Furthermore, they do not feel responsible for being unemployed, often blaming their condition on a lack of educational and financial opportunities. As one person said, "Not everyone has the same chances in life." The statement "It is not people's fault if they are poor and cannot afford a doctor" is typical. Because they feel they are not responsible for their status in life, the poor believe it is the government's responsibility to help furnish health care. They do not support, however, other actions that involve governmental subsidies, such as foreign aid. As one person said, "The government is responsible for domestic affairs and should not spend as much on foreign affairs"; another stated that "they [the government] can help people everywhere else in the world but can't help people over here." These are typical responses about the responsibilities of the federal government.

Ideally, the poor of Coberly believe that money should not be an issue in obtaining health care: "Money should not matter." All people have a right to health care and if they cannot pay for it, then they should receive it anyway. Their reason for believing the government owes them aid for health care relies heavily on two factors: (1) They have worked all their lives and often have paid Social Security taxes, or have worked a job that did not take out Social Security—work is a highly valued activity and when a person becomes elderly, he/she deserves medical services; (2) they were unable to pay Social Security taxes or were not paid equal wages for their work. As one person said, "Black people worked jobs that didn't pay Social Security and other benefits. They don't get those and it is not fair. Poor Whites and Blacks are not equal. Whites can get jobs with benefits." Because they are aware that inequalities exist in the social and economic systems, they believe that the government should help overcome these disparities by not letting people get sick or die because they are poor. Indeed, some even blame the government for these inequalities and feel that wealth should be more evenly distributed among the people. As one person put it, "A lot of problems are caused by the government. God provided enough for everyone and it should be distributed among all."

Coberly's Whites who are from the middle and upper income brackets have different beliefs and values about the role of government in the health care service delivery system. The most striking difference is the way their responses were framed. Their sentences almost always began with "if"— "if they can't pay," "if they can't afford it," "if that is the only way," and "if the distribution is controlled." Furthermore, they believe that caution should be taken in distributing aid to the poor. Indeed, many feel that only those who are not working should be helped. Their assumption is that working people actually make enough money to pay for medical care or that their insurance will pay for it. Obviously, the assumption is incorrect. Such discrepancies are not dealt with consciously by Whites and if they are forced to confront them, a kind of blaming the victim arises, such as the idea that the poor can "better themselves."

On the other hand, the Whites of Coberly believe that people should not be punished for being poor. They feel that a program such as Medicare/Medicaid should be funded but should be controlled more than it is now. They claim the widespread program is abused by doctors, which makes the cost rise. For example, statements such as (1) "government should be responsible but should not give away Food Stamps to buy beer or steaks"; (2) "more control over benefits—only to the really poor"; (3) "there are a lot of people who could work and pay their own way"; and the fear that (4) "some doctors would be abusive if government paid for care," are typical of their beliefs. Most Coberlians, however, feel that everyone is entitled to health care—especially the elderly. So the Whites, like the Blacks, feel that older people deserve and should be given the health services they need. Younger people, on the other hand, should work and pay for health services.

The effect of these expressed beliefs on behavior can be seen historically by who had access to the medical system and who did not before the passage of Medicare legislation in 1965. Upper and middle income Whites always had access and were consequently rarely, if ever, put a position of not having medical care. They do not know what it is like to be denied such care. Furthermore, their cultural model includes the basic American value correlating hard work and upward mobility. Their beliefs are then substantiated by the fact that they work hard and consequently can enjoy medical care whenever they choose to use it.

On the other hand, the poor (both Black and White) have found that working hard does not necessarily mean upward mobility or having enough money to pay for medical care. Their belief that it is not necessarily their fault that they are poor allows them to use governmental subsidies to pay for their health care. Poor Whites use the medical system more, and feel that they have more access than they did twenty years ago. Poor Blacks and some poor Whites have incorporated the choice of medical care into their repertoires only within the past two decades and, as previously discussed, younger people are then transmitted this choice. Different government policies and the beliefs of the people, however, have not led to complete medical coverage for all the people in Coberly or for all people to have access to the medical system. Coberlians' ideas about financing medical care are, however, important factors in their utilization patterns.

Summary

The variability of the health beliefs and cultural models of the people of Coberly reflect the variability of their behavior. They are the bases for the decisions Coberlians make about linking to the medical system. All these people's cultural models extend beyond the purely medical model, although all include scientific medicine as a part of their belief system. These models are transmitted to younger people who modify them to incorporate additional information from the "outside world." This process provides a better fit between these young people's behavior and their beliefs.

In this process of modification, some information is deleted and other information is added to Coberlians' cultural model. The different ethnic and income groups often have access to different information and as a consequence, their cultural models have different permutations. Among the Blacks and to some extent, the poor Whites, the use of popular medicine (teas, herbs, etc. and use of healers) is becoming less prevalent while the use of "over-the-counter medicines" and "media medicines" is increasing. Among middle and upper income Whites, the cultural model is expanding to include more "holistic" health practices. Popular medicine thus continues as a viable aspect of the health beliefs and behaviors of the people of Coberly, as does scientific medicine. They are not viewed as conflicting but as complementing one another.

People's beliefs about the medical system and how it can and cannot help them, combined with their beliefs about the causal factors of illness and healing, affect the decisions they make concerning linking to any perceived viable alternative for health care or health prevention and promotion. Knowledge of these beliefs and accompanying behaviors is important for health policy-makers and planners if they wish to increase utilization and compliance and generally to promote the health status of people in rural communities.

There are behaviors which the people of Coberly engage in even though they know these behaviors put them in high-risk categories. They may perceive the fact that they are susceptible to a disease, but they cannot change some of their behaviors such as eating certain foods. There is some kind of barrier to action. Sometimes people do not have the knowledge of lifestyle behaviors (regular exercise, low tobacco use, healthier methods of cooking, etc.) which would allow them to perceive their behaviors as high risk. Consequently, they do not perceive their susceptibility and the risks involved in specific lifestyle behaviors. Furthermore, they do not perceive the benefits to them in changing their behaviors. The perception of risk is a social process; thus, people have different preferences for risk taking (Douglas and Wildavsky 1982). People who live in different types of social structures accept certain kinds of dangers and ignore others. In Coberly, income and ethnicity are key variables in explaining people's perceptions of health risk. On the policy-making level, the risk perception process is different and, as Douglas and Wildavsky (1982) suggest, we should examine what forms of social organization are being upheld or challenged as specific risks are chosen to receive emphasis in policy making.

The people of Coberly are for the most part unaware of the macro processes that affect their health beliefs and behavior. The processes are themselves framed within a structure and an ideology which reflect the existing political economy, both private and public enterprise. Within the health system, illness becomes a social problem while the organization of illness is basically political and economic. These issues will be discussed in the following chapters.

6

Linking Community to the Health Policy System: Expanding Health Care Options

The health cultural models framed within the context of religion, family and community and manifested in the differential health behavior of the people of Coberly, are bounded and transformed by linkages to the medical system. As new health policies are implemented on the community level, people are given additional health care options. The ways in which new health services are incorporated into health behavior, while guided by beliefs, values and perceptions about health, are equally influenced by the socio-political structure that creates and implements health policies. This chapter explores how the people of Cober County linked with the health policy system to secure funds for a primary health care clinic. Exploring these linkages provides insights into the actual process and problems of policy implementation on the local level.

Securing funding for a primary health clinic in Coberly was predicated on demonstrating that the county was a medically underserved area. The people who saw the need and worked together to organize the project were concerned about the health problems in the area, particularly those of the poor. Grassroots planning required some knowledge of the political system, the relevant health policies and regulations, and people's willingness to spend a great deal of time writing proposals, working with agencies and getting the support of key local people. The history of this process in Coberly is a good example of the process of bringing change about in a small rural Southern community. It demonstrates the importance of creating linkages among systems to accomplish certain goals which function ideally to correct maladaptive aspects of the health system. In effect, the boundaries of the health care system in the county were expanded, thus more firmly establishing the dominant medical culture and structure in a traditional Southern community.

Mobilization for Change:
The Establishment of a Clinic

A citizen of Cober County for ten years, Jim Gibson worked for a social service agency, and observed the physical and mental health problems in the area daily. His concern about the people of the county, and his willingness to work for a better quality of life for them, led Mr. Gibson to serve in various leadership positions in the county and eventually to become involved in the drive to secure a primary health care clinic for the area. He was, however, always considered an "outsider" by the local people: "That yankee that moved in to town." Jane Wundram, an indigenous young woman who holds a graduate degree in social work and worked in the county for several years in a helping capacity, was, along with Jim Gibson, instrumental in developing the plans for the primary health care clinic. Joining these two in the initial stages was Sue Conboy, a person who had moved to the town four years before the development of the plans for the clinic and had immediately become active in organizing for change in the community, especially regarding the problems of the elderly. She was the director of the senior citizens center. A number of other people from local businesses and churches supported the efforts of these three, and eventually became the core of citizens that made up the clinic's board of directors. Our three major citizens, Mr. Gibson, Ms. Conboy, and Ms. Wundram, because of their jobs and ambitions, had important linkages to health-related agencies in the region and the state. They worked with district health offices and more directly with the regional Health Systems Agency and systematically worked out the necessary steps for obtaining funds from the federal government for a clinic. This collection of people can be regarded as a quasi-group. They came together for a specific action and with a specific aim or goal. Today, this group no longer exists; their goal has been accomplished. Each member had his or her own reasons for participating in the group, although the goal of their action, establishment of a clinic, was shared. Each member also had linkages to key persons in the various agencies, on all levels, whose support was needed to accomplish the goal. Each member activated these linkages during the process of planning and implementing the plans for a clinic.

According to the reflections of Jim Gibson, the first step was to organize a health fair for the county. Students from a medical school, located 60 miles away, spent a weekend at two local schools conducting screenings and dispensing information about health care. Gibson organized it so that "all social groups and all income levels could participate." The information obtained from this event indicated that there were health problems in the area of which the people were unaware. Indeed, one of the main reasons Gibson organized this fair was to make the people more aware of their health problems. The extent of such health problems was documented by surveying various workers in county agencies.

During the initial stages, Gibson was a member of the regional Health Systems Agency's board and became aware of the funds available through the Rural Health Initiative Act for establishing a clinic. The regional Health Systems Agency is a private non-profit corporation founded in 1976 for the purpose of providing effective health planning and resources development for the more than two million residents of the region. A 75 member volunteer Board of Directors, composed of both consumers and health care providers who live in the region, governs the activities of this agency. Authorized under The National Health Planning and Resources Development Act of 1974, the agency is required to develop a Health System Plan (HSP) and an Annual Implementation Plan (AIP) for the region. Ideally, the HSP is a statement by local people about their health problems and health care needs. It is a description of the region's present health status and health care system, and includes recommendations for long-range solutions that will promote improved health services and a healthful environment at a reasonable cost. The AIP identifies goals, priority objectives, and strategies as bases upon which the Resource Development Committee determines and designs specific program plans and projects. The overall development process utilizes five task forces: (1) prevention and detection, (2) primary care, (3) secondary and tertiary care, (4) environmental and occupational care, and (5) mental health, mental illness, addictive disorders and developmental disabilities. In the past few years, the HSA has been in the process of "going out of business." Its duties are being taken over by another regional planning commission.

Jim Gibson, who was, as mentioned earlier, a representative to the HSA board from Cober County, consulted with the HSA and wrote the proposal for funds for a planning grant. This was accomplished through the auspices of the Coberly Chamber of Commerce and with the technical assistance of HSA. At that time, HSA requested that DHEW designate the county a Critical Manpower Shortage Area, a prerequisite to receiving National Health Service Corps manpower or a Rural Health Initiative Grant. The Underserved Rural Area Act (HURA) is a federal grant program designed to develop comprehensive health care systems in medically needy areas. The programs may include primary care, radiology, dentistry, pharmacy services, and other specialized programs in an integrated area network of health services. The clinics result from community action and supposedly integrate their services with the existing services in the community. Thus, they become a part of the community system of medical and social services (Bernstein, et al., 1979). In referring to the Cober County grant, their publication states "the belief that every citizen in this area should have primary health care when need is a priority in the area's HSA. However, some of our residents don't have accessible or available basic care—that care delivered on out-patient basis. Efforts have been made to assure that there is a sufficient supply of qualified manpower so that everyone will have an established relationship with a primary health provider" (HSA Report 1980).

A handful of community leaders in Coberly, then, took the lead and directed the community as a whole, which Bernstein and his colleagues (1979) feel is a pioneering effort. At this point, the leaders "determined what they believed to be the best course of action and then took their case to the community for its response" (1979:20). In Coberly, these leaders elicited support from a variety of community organizations and asked specific people from many of them to serve on the board of directors.

In January 1981, HEW funded a planning grant. The clinic was incorporated by Mr. Gibson, Ms. Wundram, and Ms. Conboy in February, 1981, with the first organizational meeting occurring in March. Linda Ruhlman was hired as director. She had grown up in the area, but had lived in the upper South for several years and had worked as a health administrator in a rural clinic. She is middle-aged and dynamic, and does not identify with the residents of the county. She is, however, very perceptive about rural culture and social processes. During the three and a half years she functioned as director, she remained basically an outsider until, in the first months of 1983, she divorced her husband and married a businessman in Cober County. She is attempting to integrate into the community, although most people of Coberly still view her as an outsider.

During her first six months as director, Ms. Ruhlman created a coalition among the leaders in the county and by using the linkages already established by Mr. Gibson, Ms. Wundram and others, developed a comprehensive proposal for a health clinic. The proposal was submitted by the Board of Directors of the Cober County Primary Health Center, Inc., with Mr. Gibson as Chairperson. It states that the scope of the primary health care services will be to "provide available and accessible ambulatory care for the diagnosis and treatment of uncomplicated illnesses and disease, 24-hour coverage, minor surgery, emergency care for situations that do not require secondary or tertiary care, preventive services, case-finding services, preventive dentistry, and early periodic screening, diagnosis and treatment." In order to reach all targeted population groups, the clinic would sponsor programs of prevention and health education through educational and social service individuals, groups and systems. These services were to be integrated into a comprehensive system of health care delivery with state, federal and local agencies and programs, and with group and private practice physicians. It is believed, the proposal states, that this will ensure the clinic's "development into a financially viable, professionally attractive, and self-sustaining resource."

The overall organization of the clinic divides the personnel into an administrative section and a medical section (Figure 7). The personnel requested and subsequently funded for the clinic consist of a director, a nurse practitioner, a registered nurse, a lab technician, an executive secretary/ bookkeeper, a receptionist/medical records assistant, and an NHSC physician. The organization of the clinic, beyond the clinical staff, includes a board of directors made up of local people who represent a variety of interests in the county. In pursuit of the goal of working closely with the community, 51 percent of the initial board representation was elected by local community groups whose members were potential consumers of the medical services. The other 49 percent came from local health care providers and persons selected for their interest in the clinic and whose expertise is in the health and/or management areas. Specific areas of knowledge and competency within the board of directors include the groups listed in Table 15.

The services required by HEW are the ones which the clinic personnel emphasize as the major needs of the population. Since a systematic needs assessment survey had not been conducted in Cober County, the needs reported in the grant proposal were based on the health status indicators of the county and the minimal nature of health services there. The clinic's services proposal included: (1) family planning, with special emphasis on adolescent patients and screening exams; (2) well-adult care, with the main objectives being prevention, early detection and patient education, and the establishment of linkages with health advocacy agencies and organizations (i.e., Red Cross Society); (3) periodic screening for diseases known to be prevalent in the population (hypertension, diabetes, cancer, tuberculosis) and a component of the ongoing health program; (4) well-child care, focusing on prevention of childhood diseases through immunization and early detection of health problems through exams; (5) prenatal care to pregnant women, with emphasis on adolescent patients and linkages to other agencies; (6) chronic disease care aimed at alleviating the degenerative effects of chronic disease through accessible medical management by providing individual treatment of patients; (7) hypertension (a major problem in Cober County) treatment through blood pressure monitoring; (8) preventive dental care to assess the need for a dentist in the county and to provide linkages to dental resources; (9) emergency medical services provided by medical personnel on a rotating basis; (10) a nutritional program designed to improve people's nutritional status (Indeed, the latter is a crucial need in the county. Over 40 percent of school age children participate in the free lunch program

148

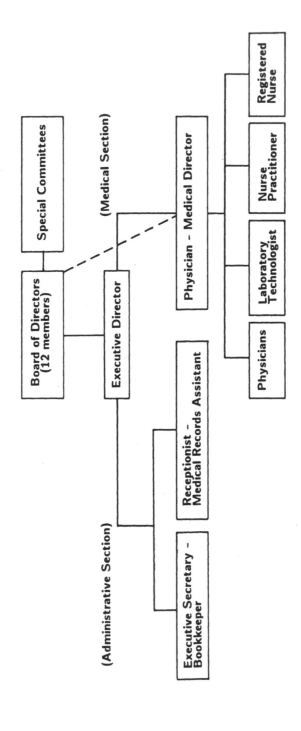

Figure 7. Organization of Cober County Primary Health Care Center, Inc.

TABLE 15
Composition of Board of Directors of Cober County PHCC (1982)

Consumers	Race/Sex
Lions Club representative—fund raising, health need identification and development of preventive/remedial service, business management	W/M
National Association for the Advancement of Colored People representative—community organization, equal opportunity advocacy, individual rights, needs of economically disadvantaged	B/M
Association for Retarded Citizens representative—fund raising, needs and rights of the handicapped, voluntary organization relationships	W/F
Town Councils—local, state and federal laws, regulations, resources, and contact persons	W/M
Retired Teachers Association representative—needs of elderly persons on limited incomes, sources of contacts with influential local and state personages	W/F
Voters League representative—rights, needs, and procedures of residents assuring fair representation and receipt of services	B/F

Other Representatives	
Chamber of Comerce representative—needs of local industry and community businesses, responsible and effective management practices	W/M
County Commissioners representative—local, state, and federal laws, resources, administrative guidelines, and influential contacts	W/F
CAP-Nutrition/Senior Citizens representative—medical and nutritional needs of the elderly, preventive methods of health care	W/F
Public Health Department R.N.—health needs of residents, preventive and curative medical care, regional and state health resources and contact persons, rural health techniques	W/F
Educational Systems representative—knowledge of health needs of the youth in the area, teaching techniques	B/M
Dr. D. L. Jones is providing medical expertise and technical advice in the development of the facility design, staffing pattern, on-site services, and physician review and selection for the PHCC. Dr. Jones is a general practitioner in Upson County, on staff at Upson Memorial Hospital, and on the Credentials Committee of said hospital. Dr. Jones' father practiced medicine in Cober County for 35 years, hence Dr. Jones' interest in the development of an efficient and responsible practice to serve Cober County residents.	W/M

Source: Regional Health Systems Agency, Inc., Statistical Profile, 1980.

and at least 640 elderly persons in the county have been identified as needing one nutritional meal per day. There are serious problems with obesity, anemia and malnutrition.); (11) health education in the areas of prevention, maintenance and treatment (including well-child, well-adolescent, well-adult, acute episodic and chronic disease); (12) transportation—only a moderate problem except for the elderly and persons who are home-bound due to their physical condition—to be coordinated with the senior citizens' center; (13) social services in the county used as linkages to social service agencies in the area to improve the health status of a patient by, for example, helping him/her to enroll in Medicaid; (14) supplemental services as required for diagnostic laboratory procedures; (15) specialty medical consultation in adjacent counties, to be used when a patient needs special medical attention; (16) the utilization of hospitals in adjacent counties when patients need hospitalization; (17) pharmacy services, to be coordinated with physician services to increase patient accessibility; (18) home health care services, to be coordinated with the clinic physician (an estimated 92 persons have need of these services, according to the Area Planning and Development Commission) and with (19) extended care facilities (an estimated 130 elderly persons in the county need such services, again according to the Area Planning and Development Commission); (20) evaluation procedures, to be implemented in order to determine whether or not the clinic is meeting its objectives. These procedures do not include any extensive external review process.

A majority of the clinic's potential patients were thought to be either poor or below the poverty level. Thus, it was projected that 13 percent would pay by Medicare, 8 percent by Medicaid, 13 percent of people below the poverty level by direct pay, 33 percent through Medicare, and 33 percent pay in full at the time of services. It was assumed that perhaps only 80 percent of direct pay fees would be collected. So far, however, the majority of the users are Medicare and Medicaid patients and poor patients, with the middle-class patients continuing to use their established physician in another county.

Problems of Implementation

Funding for the clinic was approved in July of 1981, and the director began to hire staff and to have the building chosen for the clinic remodeled (on the square in Coberly). The planning process followed, more or less, the major phases of facility development as outlined by Alford (1979). They are: (1) planning and programming, (2) schematic design, (3) design development, (4) construction documentation, (5) bidding and negotiation, (6) construction administration and (7) post-construction documentation and evaluation. The phase of bidding and negotiation was not as extensive as it perhaps could have been, since the contractor was a part of the friendship/ kinship network of one of the major supporters of the clinic in the community. Administering the construction phase was difficult for Ms. Ruhlman. According to her, the construction workers were unaccustomed to taking orders from a woman and generally ignored her directions. The contractors did not build the rooms to specifications, went above the estimated cost, and took more time than they had anticipated. Eventually, they were fired and new builders were hired to attempt to rectify the problems with clinic construction. Finally, the building was completed, several months past the initial deadline.

Another problem arose in attempting to hire local people for clinic personnel positions. According to the board, there simply were not any qualified people who understood the procedures involved in beginning and operating a clinic. An executive secretary, Ms. Reed, was hired and along with the director handled all the administrative, construction and personnel problems. Again, Ms. Reed had problems relating to the construction workers, and they, at times, would have rather heated discussions about the design of the rooms, quality of materials, etc. So, not only were the two women and the construction workers caught in a cultural conflict, the two women were "outsiders" and, as such, were thought to be unaware of how to deal with construction matters of any kind. These problems persisted with both sets of contractors, although the construction company that finished the building was more amenable to working with Ms. Ruhlman and Ms. Reed.

The most difficult problem was, however, finding a physician. A majority of the medical schools with programs in primary health care were contacted with few or no results. The salary of $50,000 was funded through NHSC and the practice was virtually guaranteed. The lack of interest in the position surprised the people of Coberly since they felt that their town and county were attractive and good places to live. Furthermore, the town is located within 60 miles of a major city in the South with all the recreational and artistic resources of most larger cities. These resources were described in a letter and flyer that were sent several times to medical schools. Still, over a year passed before a physician was hired for the clinic.

In the meantime, Ms. Ruhlman decided to open the clinic with a nurse practitioner (NP) and a registered nurse (RN). The NP was recruited from the city, while the RN was a native of the area. The clinic opened in January of 1982, although the renovation of the building had not been completed. A physician in a nearby town was hired for one afternoon a week. Otherwise, the NP and RN handled the health problems of the patients. They immediately began to implement community health programs by making connections with other services in the area. They especially cooperated with the public health clinic programs creatively run by an energetic young RN. Two of the programs of particular importance were the family planning program and the nutritional program. Another strong linkage was to the senior citizens' center with its emphasis on nutritional education and, to a lesser degree, the home extension services in the county, again headed by a creative young woman who emphasized the community and rural development component of the program. Together these groups developed a diabetic support group and an obesity support group (two of the major contributors to hypertension). They reported, however, that it was difficult to get people to attend these meetings and, as of the writing of this book, they have failed to attract enough people to justify the continuance of the groups. Another factor that has caused problems for these innovative programs is that the NP and the RN from the public health clinic left the area within the first year of operation of the primary health care clinic, thus reducing even further the small amount of support the clinic was receiving from the community. Continuity was lost.

In the Fall of 1982, a physician was hired by the clinic—Dr. Lin, from Taiwan. He was trained in a medical school in California and had worked for a few years in the upper South. He moved into Coberly with his family and planned to settle there for a long time. The number of visits to the clinic increased upon his arrival, many of the people we interviewed reporting that they liked Dr. Lin and planned to continue to use him as their physician. That same Fall the nurse practitioner left for a city job. She was not replaced for over a year. Dr. Lin and Ms. Ruhlman felt that a NP was not really needed. The director stated that "The physician, at this point, can take care of the clientele." With this decision, the services of the clinic became more clinically oriented and less preventive oriented.

In 1984, Dr. Lin left the clinic and after four months was replaced by Dr. Young, a white middle class Southerner who immediately became a part of the community power structure. His ambition and need for control of the clinic led to a severe conflict with Ms. Ruhlman. They accused one another of unethical conduct and, mysteriously, some of the crucial records that would clear up the conflict turned up missing. Because Dr. Young had, in a short time, been able to gain the support of the Board of Directors, Ms. Ruhlman was forced to resign in 1985. A replacement has not been appointed and, according to clinic personnel, the position will not be filled by anyone other than Dr. Young, who took over those duties. At present, the support groups and outreach programs are not functioning. Linkages with other services in the area have decreased. The number of visits by patients has increased over the years, and since the outreach program that brought about an important level of accessibility for the chronically ill has disappeared, the clinic is basically a secondary level facility rather than a primary care facility. It does not provide most of the services required in its mandate.

Community Issues and Problems

Not surprisingly, almost 40 percent of our sample in Coberly was unaware either that a clinic existed in the community or that it was open for business. A majority had little or no knowledge of the efforts to establish a clinic and 20 percent felt that a clinic was not needed in the town. Almost everyone interviewed had his or her own physician and most had little difficulty in visiting them. Most said that it was only a 15 or 20 minute ride to their physician and that they would continue to see him. Part of this decision was based on their experiences with physicians in the community over the past two decades. Many felt that if they did change physicians and use the clinic in Coberly, there was a chance that the clinic physician might leave, and then they would have a difficult time getting their present physician to accept them back, especially since they believe that many of the physicians in the area do not accept new patients. Others expressed concern about breaking trust with their current doctor and said that if they needed to go back to him or her, they would not be welcomed. Reasoning from these assumptions, over 25 percent stated that they would not utilize the clinic except in cases of emergencies.

Generally, the people who were aware of the processes involved in establishing a clinic were middle class and, again, a majority of them said that they would not use the clinic. Most, however, felt that the clinic was needed for the poor and they thus supported its establishment. They felt that a need existed with the poor people and that the clinic would be a "welfare clinic." We found that some of the leaders of the community did not support the establishment of a health clinic; they felt that it was "pushed by outsiders for their own purposes"—in other words, that it was not a true community effort but an effort on the part of a few for mostly economic or political gains. One person said "everyone here has a doctor and can get any kind of medical help they need. We don't need to spend money on a clinic in Coberly." Another person stated that the support came from people who thought they would "make money on the construction and the renting of the building." There is consequently little consensus among Coberlians on the need for and usefulness of the clinic. One year after it was opened, many continued to say that they would not use its resources.

Another rather serious community issue that continues today involves the relationship between the primary health care clinic and the public health clinic. Ideally, their functions should overlap very little; in reality, for the first year there was a considerable overlapping of the services they provided, especially since the primary health care clinic was not staffed by a physician initially. Thus, the staffs of both the clinics cooperated and developed mutual programs. In the beginning, there was a great deal of interaction between them, both formally and informally. Presently, this is no longer the case for several reasons.

The public health nurse took a leave of absence and was not immediately replaced. Several members of the Health Board informally recommended to the District Health Office that the public health clinic be closed. They said that with the primary health care clinic in the community, there was really no need for the public health clinic. Not surprisingly, two of these people were strong supporters of the establishment of the primary health clinic. Other citizens of the county argued that the public health clinic was needed, especially by the poor who could not pay for services at the primary health clinic. Thus, closing it would limit their access to health services. The latter contingent won the argument and the public health clinic was not closed. A local nurse was assigned to operate it, although several services were deleted from its activities. In addition, neither the physician, NP or RN at the primary health clinic had met the new public health nurse six months after these changes.

From my interviewing and observations, it appears that the cooperative nature of the relationship between the two clinics is subsiding and that both staffs are aware of a competition for patients, as well as an overlapping of activities. As previously mentioned, coordinating records is a problem. Perhaps more seriously, the new public health nurse has a different perspective and training from the previous one. She is well organized and caring about the patients but goes strictly "by the book" and is proud of the order one finds in the clinic. She is not, however, innovative or particularly interested in developing service programs with the primary health care clinic. Indeed, she had never met the personnel of the primary health care clinic after being in her job several months and after two years, she was still unfamiliar with most of the personnel.

As a consequence of the perceived competition and different approaches to health care, a schism has developed between the clinics, with potentially serious consequences for the people of Cober County. With funds for the public health clinic shrinking and the state level decision-makers looking to close clinics that are no longer economically feasible, the clinic in Coberly was targeted as a possible liability at the time of this study. Furthermore, the federal government's new approach to funding—block grants—is causing major problems for state and local health officials. The state has taken a major responsibility for the primary health care clinic, creating a rather ironic situation: it is responsible for both clinics. In 1986, both clinics are still operating, with the public health nurse making referrals to the doctor when she feels it is necessary. The clinics do not cooperate on health programs that reach out to the community, since the primary health care clinic has none.

Policy Issues and Problems

Additional problems encountered during the implementation phase of the primary health care clinic concerned the policy system. On the local level, only a city license was required, while there were no regulations on the state level beyond the procedures involved with Medicare. Since it was initially funded by the federal government, the guidelines of the Department of Health and Human Services were followed in establishing the clinic. Several of the problems in establishing and maintaining a rural clinic stem from the assumptions made in these general regulations about such clinics.

According to all the policy-makers I interviewed, the regulations are based on urban criteria and measurements. In order to establish an effective clinic with rural access, there must be linkages to hospitals, mental health facilities, a pharmacy, and other health facilities/agencies. The regulations, however, do not take into account time demands on a physician in isolated rural areas. For example, the regulations state that emergency rooms cannot be used for backup and that the clinic must have 24-hour coverage. This assumes that more than one physician will be close by in the area or work for the clinic. Thus, a clinic with only one physician must keep him/her on call 24 hours; this makes it difficult to find a physician because he/she must be willing to commit himself/herself to a very demanding job.

HHS regulations also require that a physician have hospital privileges; again, this is thought to be an urban-based policy by my respondents. In rural areas, however, the physician may be a long distance from a hospital and the regulations limit such a distance. All my respondents stated that many problems would be solved if the regulations converted the distance restrictions into the time it would take to travel. In addition, conflicts have arisen between hospital and clinic. Some hospitals, which are in control of this linkage, either refuse or make it difficult for an "outside physician" to acquire privileges. They feel the expense to the hospital will overshadow the advantages of adding another physician to their staff.

In their section on community acceptance, Bernstein et al. (1979) feel that before the leadership of a community fans out across the community to present the idea of a new health practitioner clinic, they "must have a good idea of what aspects of the program they should discuss with potential supporters. Will the administrator of the nearby hospital be impressed with the possibility of attracting more doctors to the area? Will the hospital board members want to know that the hospital can expect additional refunds . . . ? Will the county commission have a new health resource to turn to when they try to attract growth and industry to the area?" (1979:30). Furthermore, will other institutions like schools, churches, businesses and individuals such as pharmacists and nearby doctors view the new clinic as a resource or a threat? As far as I was able to ascertain in Coberly, the leaders mainly stayed within the county and made very little effort to elicit the support of nearby hospitals and physicians (all outside the county). Consequently, problems arose with these forces outside the county that reflected a difference in ideology. Doctors in nearby hospitals told the director of the primary health care clinic in Coberly that they did not support the idea of a primary health clinic and resented the use of the "taxpayer's money" to build a clinic that was not needed. Furthermore, they were reluctant to give a "foreign doctor" permission to utilize the services of their hospitals. As a consequence, we find that in Coberly problems in activating linkages of the health system, as suggested in the policy guidelines, slowed down or precluded restructuring the system of health care.

Another problem with the regulations, according to my survey, involves the requirement that a utilized pharmacy must be within a certain distance of the clinic. This makes the cost of medicines dependent upon what the local pharmacy charges, thus the patients potentially may have to pay more than is necessary. This suppresses competition since in rural areas, like Cober County, there is only one pharmacy. The requirement that a clinic has to pay a provider for any services also creates problems with establishing linkages between agencies. The public health department and the mental health agencies are specifically mentioned as necessary linkages, yet there are problems with payment to providers as well as with record keeping. Although referrals are constantly being made, the administrators are finding it difficult to share patient records. If the patient goes to the public health department, often the records are not returned to the primary health care clinic, making the clinic reporting to HHS appear to have fewer patients than it actually has at any one time.

Two additional problems involve regulations that the local administrators in Coberly feel again are biased toward urban areas. Projects under $200,000 cannot be represented in the Health and Human Services review. Most rural health grants are under this amount and, as a consequence, the rural projects are underrepresented during times of decision-making at the regional or national levels. Another potential problem involves the requirement that a written support statement from the local AMA secretary must accompany a refunding request. In the Coberly area, this organization has not completely supported the establishment of a clinic or aided in finding a physician for the clinic. Indeed, my respondents feel that American Medical Association members see the primary health care clinic as being in competition with their services and that they only reluctantly support its functioning.

The director of the senior citizens' center discussed similar problems with the regulations under which her center operated. Overall, the problems of distance and time in rural areas are quite different from the same problems in urban areas, a factor she felt is not considered when health policies are constructed. For example, there is a restriction on the number of miles of van use which was exceeded by just picking up the participants in her program. There may be five miles between people's houses, so the average monthly van use mileage and time generally far exceeded the amounts prescribed. In addition, these restrictions preclude taking the elderly to programs/activities in nearby towns and, because the state vehicle has to be utilized on all official trips, the cost was higher than if they took an automobile. Another regulation states that meals taken to houses must be delivered within 20 minutes. This was impossible in several cases because the recipients lived more than 20 minutes away from the center; as a consequence, they did not receive the meals. Lastly, the cost of and time spent in identifying the needy is greater in rural areas although the regulations are the same for both rural and urban areas. The director of the senior citizens' center felt that these problems were the result of policies made at the state or federal level with little or no knowledge of the unique problems of delivering services in rural areas.

Even on the state level, policies do not differentiate between rural and urban environments. Several people I interviewed on this level, in contrast to the local level, stated that they had never thought about making a distinction and after thinking about my questions about the unique problems of rural areas, all were able to delineate "rural" as a unique problem to solve. Most said that they attempt to deal with key target (high-risk) populations in each county, with rurality not being one of the variables considered in their planning and policy process. The issues and concerns the state level policymakers reported generally related to administration and cost. All agreed that the cost of delivering health care in rural areas is higher and the contact rate per dollar is low. Because of this, some felt that urban areas have been favored in allocating resources. As a consequence, fewer people have access to health facilities which, of course, accounts for the fact that even though rural people are poorer than urban people, their rate of reimbursement for health services through Medicare and Medicaid is lower than that of the poor in urban areas.

The administration of state services is somewhat different in rural areas. The regions are larger and the staffs smaller. One respondent stated that "in rural areas people are making decisions (often about health care) who should not be making them." In contrast, local people feel that state people should not be making so many decisions which affect their functions in delivering services. Another problem state level people are concerned with involves linking local clinics to hospitals (secondary and tertiary care). In urban areas, the development of linkages through referral systems is a relatively easy process. In rural areas, however, it is more difficult for the providers as well as the consumers. Compliance then becomes a major problem. Overall, rural people are less dependent on the mainstream health care system than those in urban areas and, as a consequence, they have fewer resources or no resources to turn to, which accounts for the lower health status of rural people.

In 1977, a new thrust was initiated in the state to reallocate resources in support of primary health care. Grants were obtained to train nurse practitioners and public health nurses to work with community leaders and to assess the need for health services in the state's counties. Furthermore, this initiative emphasized helping counties become certified for NHSC. According to the director of the Coberly clinic, two-thirds of the cases that go to emergency rooms in the state are primary health problems, so "many people are not getting into the system at the right end." He sees his tasks as building primary health care systems and linkages via referral systems to other forms of care. The emphasis should be on prevention, a goal everyone at the state level acknowledges.

All the policymakers and planners interviewed felt that the major health service problem in rural areas is personnel distribution. The key issue is how to attract physicians to rural areas. Studies conducted on the maldistribution of physicians have shown that there are several factors involved in making decisions to locate in urban areas. The most important ones are educational and cultural opportunities, money, and the wishes of their spouses. In the past several years, several policy alternatives have been suggested to rectify the maldistribution problem. Presently, however, there are no overall national policies that provide incentives for physicians to practice in rural areas. As a consequence, national and state level health personnel feel that paraprofessionals such as nurse practitioners and physician's assistants are the answer to distributing medical personnel in rural areas.

The Failure of Primary Health Care in Coberly

The health behavior of the people of Coberly is structured by the traditional and institutional service options available to them. The institutional options are the health policies which are, in turn, structured by the sociopolitical and ideological structure of the society, the topic of the following chapters. The primary health care clinic in Coberly is a product of a specific health care policy, and has failed to meet objectives of the policy.

In 1979, Davis and Marshall identified three alternative systems of health care in the rural South. They are: (1) primary health care, (2) group health practices, and (3) comprehensive health centers. To evaluate the effectiveness of these alternatives, Walker (1978) collected data on a sample of health care delivery systems in the rural South. She found that the primary health care models work well in small rural places where it is difficult to support a physician or which cannot attract a physician. The PHC clinics are generally non-profit and employ one or two primary health practitioners (nurse practitioners, physician's assistants and nurse midwives) and a part-time physician. The second model, the group health practice, is viable in communities with a population of 6,000-20,000. This model has two or three physicians working as a team with primary practitioners and employs dentists, provides laboratory and emergency facilities and has a professional manager. The third model, the comprehensive health center, works well in areas of high poverty but is quite expensive—$1 million to $3 million per year. It depends on large grants to supplement insurance reimbursement and local resources. Because of its wide range of services, Walher found that this model dramatically affects the health status of a community.

National health policy divides PHC services into four basic categories. They are: (1) Primary Preventive Services, including family planning, prenatal care, well child care, well adolescent care, well adult care, preventive dental services, health education and nutrition services; (2) Secondary Preventive Services, including periodic screening for the entire population, acute episodic medical care and management of chronic medical problems; (3) Support Services, including translation, laboratory services, diagnostic x-ray, pharmacy services, specialty and subspecialty medical consultation, hospitalization and transportation and (4) Supplemental Health Services, including dental diagnostic and treatment services, mental health services, social services, crippled children's services, nursing home services, emerging medical services and environmental health services (U.S. Department of HEW, 1980). Primary health care offers crucial and viable options in communities such as Coberly and can affect the health order of a community if (1) it is comprehensive and provides health care rather than just medical care and (2) it is established in a participatory fashion, including the results of research on the community: its components, and its level of health need and organization (Sheps, et al., n.d.).

Primary health care options do not exist in Coberly even four years after the clinic opened its doors. In fact, as previously stated, the few outreach programs that were attempted in the initial months failed. The nurse practitioner at the clinic in 1986 stated that "we have no preventive programs that reach out into the community." The clinic functions basically as an outpatient diagnostic and treatment center. Most of the people who utilize the clinic do so either for acute health problems such as colds, flu, and other common ailments of adults and children, or prenatal and postnatal care, chronic problems—mostly of the elderly—and general checkups. There are no dental services, and the only health education is done through consultation with the nurse practitioner or the doctor. None of the other services designated by the national PHC policy is in operation; nor does the clinic have community input except via the board of directors, all members of which are now upper-income Whites.

In rural areas generally, many of these services are unavailable to people, and the categorization of these services is often rather arbitrary. For example, classifying mental health as a supplemental service demonstrates the assumptions of the biomedical system in separating mental and physical health. Furthermore, the services are generally planned with little or no input from the community in terms of organizational structures that will fit the community and with little or no research on the appropriate levels of intervention and the corresponding services which are needed, as in the case of Coberly.

The PHC clinic is providing an option to the people of Coberly, but it is one that does not address itself to many of their needs. It does not expand the cultural knowledge of the people beyond the model. It does provide services that aid in the process of medicalization (to be discussed in Chapter 8), particularly of the poor and elderly, and it upholds the health beliefs of the few upper-income Whites who use it. It links people to a medical system that designs and implements services that are superimposed on the community of Coberly, with pitifully little knowledge about its culture and social systems.

Rural primary health care services should vary according to the needs of the specific community, and should be based on the social/cultural system of the community, the health risks of the people (based on epidemiological data) and their ability to pay for the needed services. Once these factors have been delineated, the needed PHC services should be prioritized and integrated with existing services and resources in the community through the organizing actions of people from the entire hierarchy of the health system. What happened in Coberly is an example of what results from mobilizing some of the people in the community and setting priorities that uphold the sociopolitical system in which PHC policies are made. Although the clinic is successful in providing outpatient treatment, it is not successful in providing preventive services. This failure is due to a number of factors, all of which can be understood by examining the cultural and social systems of policymakers. On one level, it may appear that lack of money, personnel and time are the reasons such services cannot be delivered. To understand their explanations of why there is not enough time, money or personnel, the systems of explanation and the belief systems of health policymakers must be examined. While they leave out a critical element in their planning—the cultural and social system of the people—community studies often leave out a cultural description of the macrolevel: the institutions that impinge on the community. This level will be explored in the next chapter.

7

Health Policy
as a Cultural System

Culture and Policy

Social, economic and political structures create and limit the health possibilities of a population. They produce and reproduce medical knowledge by transmitting information to people about the dominant health care system. Like the cultural system of the people of Coberly, whose symbols of health provide meaning to them, and which bound their behavioral choices, a cultural component also confers meaning upon the policy system's structure and functions and bounds the possibilities for health policy. It is at this macrolevel, that of the structure and culture of the health policy system, that linkages are made with the population of a community. Both levels affect the formulation, planning, and implementation of health policy on the local level. In this chapter, I will discuss health policy as a cultural system that provides guidelines for instituting behavioral and structural changes in the health system. I argue that culture mediates (constitutes and is constituted by) health policies and how they are formulated and carried out. A cultural approach can explain why there is not enough money, time and personnel to implement all the parts of a PHC program in Coberly. In this chapter, I will first describe the policy process and the key symbols used by policy-makers to create frames that define health problems and delineate solutions to these problems. I will emphasize rural health care in examining the major metaphors or cultural models actualized by policy-makers to create the policy system. Finally, I will discuss how the policy systems interface with social science to give meaning to the symbolic process of policy-making.

The policy process is a system of multilayered "webs of significance" which convey meaning to the actions of people involved in developing, making and implementing policy. It has a structure (for action) that can be understood on one hand within the framework of a hierarchical systems approach and, on the other hand, as an ideology (meanings) that governs the choice of policies within the repertoire of possible policies. These are two sides of the same coin, and analyzing one without an understanding of the other distorts the meaning of the processes of change in health policy.

Cultural models are the coherent framework within which selected facts are ordered and related. When applied to social policies, the main function of a cultural model is to guide policy construction by ordering and organizing certain facts into causal theories which then specify appropriate policy interventions. Because they include problem definitions and the ordering of what is considered relevant and valid knowledge, the models limit intervention choices by systematically excluding consideration of alternative frameworks (or interventions). In this sense, models can take on the character of ideologies in addition to reflecting an ideology. Thus, "existing institutional and power relationships are maintained by a policy paradigm that imposes problem definitions that legitimate the rationalization (through planning) and reorganization (through coordination) of existing services" (Estes 1979:5).

Indeed, social phenomena cannot be understood in isolation from the ideology which organizes evidence, interprets it and implies policy decisions which are consistent with it. Policy and knowledge measured by social scientists are interactive; as policy changes, "knowledge is used selectively to qualify action reached on other grounds" (Rein 1976:34). Furthermore, "policy paradigms change in response to social, economic and political changes—that is, they change because they have to rationalize a different reality, not because research has revealed that the interpretation of earlier circumstances was wrong" (Rein 1976:110). The meaning of these changing realities is a product of collective experiences which transcend the individual experience yet encompass all individuals. Policy paradigms become metaphors of how a particular social phenomenon works, and permit policymakers to reason from the familiar to the unfamiliar, thus creating new frames. "Familiar concepts are brought into unfamiliar situations and in the process they transform the unfamiliar into the familiar" (Rein 1979:75).

During the past two decades, American society has experienced dramatic shifts in societal norms and in the process, many current issues of society, such as equity of services to all minority groups, have been translated into social policies that make up a system and into symbols which provide meaning to the social change processes. Reich (1985) has labeled this process "public philosophy," a set of assumptions and logical links by which we interpret and integrate social reality, conveyed through parables and made manifest in the stories we tell about events. A public philosophy informs our sense of what our society is about, what it is for (1985:68).

The Process of Policy Construction

Policy construction follows a "critical path": critical in the sense that it affects the lives and experiences of people in American society by structuring parts of their behavior and providing meaning to their experiences within the political economy. The cultural system includes a system of symbols that, although changing, structures the reality of individuals in the health system. There is present in American society today a general model of the policy process that provides an order to the health behavior and beliefs of health care consumers as well as policymakers. These groups share a set of metaphors which guide behavior and seemingly avert the perils of chaos in the midst of social change. These are the metaphors policymakers live by (Lakoff & Johnson 1980) and use to make sense out of our health world. The metaphors used in the health field are generative in that they "carry over" from one domain of experience to another (Schon 1979); a kind of reasoning by analogy from other systems in the society. The process involved in policy construction utilizes generic metaphors for interpreting how health problems are defined (framed) and for identifying the possible solutions to these perceived problems in the health policy world. During this process, problems are framed in new ways and new solutions are generated; details of this part of the process will be examined later in this chapter.

Social policy is generally considered a problem-solving enterprise, although Schon (1979) feels that it is more of a problem-setting enterprise. It has " . . . more to do with ways in which we frame the purposes to be achieved than with the selection of optimal means for achieving them" (1979:255). The delineations of health problems by policymakers and planners are based on "stories" people tell, or as Schon says "stories people tell about troublesome situations—stories in which they describe what is wrong and what needs fixing" (1979:255). The bases for constructing these problems are the metaphors underlying the stories. For example, the "problem" of providing secondary or tertiary care in rural areas can be "solved" by linkages to urban areas. This problem and its solution are bounded by the "linkage" and "high tech" metaphors that generated the problem in the first place, with the underlying meaning of secondary and tertiary care as a necessary service for all people, but one that is not important enough to provide in rural areas. The solution then, is to link the rural health system to urban service, and consequently, to transport rural people to urban centers. Obviously, this solution is generated from the metaphor, and its underlying assumption which guides policy is to keep the health power in urban areas. I am not implying that this is a bad policy; it is just one possibility for constructing a meaningful health order in our society.

Of course, conflicting frames can be generated, leading to debates over the different and often contradictory frames. In the process of health policy construction, frames are restructured and new metaphors generated, often with very little reliance on empirical research. These frames, once named, help policymakers redirect their attention to what they believe to be the key variables of and solutions to a health problem. They also give the selected variables a coherent organization that not only describes what is wrong but also provides a probable solution. Thus, policymakers make a "normative leap from data to recommendations, from fact to values, from 'is' to 'ought'" (Rein & Schon 1977). In this process, some variables are selected as relevant, often as causal agents of the problem, and other variables are left out and ignored. The basis for this selection depends on the key metaphors, and their underlying assumptions about the nature of reality itself (what is), and what is thus considered normative. The policy process— its development, implementation and evaluation—is basically an interaction, a communication based on language and the meaning that is passed among groups of people, the values that are held by a group of people and the action that comes from the exchange of messages and values. Within this process, problems are framed and solutions sought based on the slice of reality that is deemed relevant to the problem. The problems delineate priorities in the policy process which in turn set up the policy agendas of all those involved, including the legislative and executive branches of government, lobbyists, policy analysts and special interest groups. All these groups frame the problems slightly differently, have both public and hidden agendas (often conflicting metaphors), and feel that a specific health problem is legitimate and their solution feasible.

Health policies can originate from all or any of these groups but whatever their source, all must go through the political process. This "makes" the policy as distinguished from administering or implementing it. The makers can be from the legislative, the executive or the judicial branch of government on either the federal or state level. This public sector ideally makes policies for the "public good," a judgement generally based on the political metaphors which frame the problems and solutions. The "private sector," on the other hand, consists of a variety of interest groups ranging from large business corporations to organizations based on ethnicity, class or sex. These groups/ organizations have a variety of motives for restructuring health policies and base their desired changes on metaphors which often incorporate conflicting assumptions and beliefs that are never really resolved but are functional in that they relieve tensions at a particular point through superficial compromises (ambiguous symbols).

Health Policy Metaphors

Health policy metaphors are reflected in the language used in the policy arena. Edelman states that "it is through metaphor, metonymy and syntax that linguistic references evoke mystic cognitive structures in people's minds" (1977:16). Furthermore, he feels that metaphors can become myths, such as the metaphor of "underserved area" which guides health policies in rural areas. Based on the syntax of a sentence, the entire structure of belief and meaning is evoked and becomes more powerful. It is thus the form of the policymakers' statements that often transmits messages which influence public opinion, not necessarily the content (Edelman 1971, 1977).

In the past few years, several groups with conflicting metaphors have affected health policies. One of the dominant metaphors in the 1960s was "health is a right," a frame that was picked up by the World Health Organization. The belief underlying this metaphor is that health can be used to restructure inequality in the social system. Equality is valued as good, while inequality is bad. Consequently, other variables, such as cost effectiveness, must be cut out of the policy frame in order to redistribute health care services in both urban and rural areas, with consumers having a major role in decision-making.

Another guiding metaphor in health policy construction which may or may not support the belief in "health is a right" is that of "market reform." Paradoxically, two opposing factions use this frame to bound their policies. Some groups feel that "more of everything" will solve health problems, i.e., more doctors, more drugs, more clinics, etc. One of the underlying assumptions of this paradigm is a support of professional expansion, and professional monopoly and dominance over the health care delivery system. Furthermore, the provider and not the consumer is in control, resulting in a restructuring based on the values of the medical profession. Another faction under the market reformers' spell believes that "more is better" as long as the market demands it. This laissez faire approach likewise assumes control of the medical profession over decisions on distribution of services and that the consumers will only demand (need?) what they can afford.

A third metaphor that arose out of the 1970s is that of "rational management," i.e., restructuring the system so that health managers are in control, rather than the consumers or providers. Ideally, both consumers and providers will affect decision-making, but the organization and administration of the health system is most valued. It is assumed that this solution to the delivery of health services prevents unorganized service delivery through controlled planning, thus solving problems through coordination of resources and services. It is also assumed that rational management based on cost efficiency will contain and lower the cost of health care services. In recent years, this metaphor has been activated through increasing control by corporations (Starr 1984).

Most recent policy priorities utilize these metaphors to guide problem-setting. According to Fein (1980), the recent issues in health policy construction are: (1) cost containment, (2) human capital (manpower problems and solutions), (3) equity versus efficiency, (4) federal governmental control, (5) the structure of health insurance, (6) health planning, and (7) health as a right. All of these issues are shaped by particular economic and political values, all of which are represented in both the public and private sectors of policymaking. The result of these contradictory frames is apparent confusion and the lack of an organized health policy in U.S. society.

What is apparent, however, may not be real within a broader metaphor's structure or level of explanation. When viewed within the syntactic structure of democracy and capitalism, a meaningful system emerges. Policy is pluralistic and incremental; policy changes move slowly and piecemeal. Health policy appears to be a patchwork quilt with little patterning, but allowing all factions to compete for power. The assumption here is that all groups have equal access to the policymakers. Experience has demonstrated, however, that groups (public or private) with more money and organization have more influence on policymaking, and that the result is the creation of overspecific policies which address the needs and concerns of one part of the health system to the neglect of another. This process fits the dominant values of the political economy which controls the policy process in American society, since it incorporates contradictory beliefs about how to restructure society in general and health policy in particular. Each group has specific guiding metaphors that fit its syntax (liberal or conservative). These "multiple realities," as Edelman calls them, are threatened by opposing metaphors. And as we shall examine in the next section, there is no definitive way of verifying or falsifying the other group's beliefs. Obviously, these contradictory beliefs provide for alternative worldviews on an issue, but, as in the "closed predicament" as defined by Robin Horton (1967), alternative causal agents and solutions to problems are a threat to the established, dominant body of knowledge. These alternative views taken together (an open predicament?) allow the health system to change and feed into other systems (economy, religion) in a society, depending on the prevalence of the key metaphor at any point.

Policy alternatives are delineated by the public and private sectors through policy analysis of health problems in order to determine the "best" change within their worldview. According to Ukeles (1977) policy analysis should: (1) assess the policymaking environment within which the analyst and the relevant decisionmakers are operating, (2) identify policy questions or problems needing resolutions, (3) identify policy alternatives appropriate to policymaking environments, (4) identify criteria relevant to choosing alternatives and (5) assess pros and cons of each alternative in terms of relevant criteria. These relevant criteria, of course, are based on the guiding metaphors generated by the belief in proper intersections of the health system with other systems of the society, intersections which the analysts believe will provide the best restructuring of society and create a better health order.

Rural Health Frames in the U.S.:
Rural Versus Urban

The construction of a rural health reality includes in its frames the physical handicaps of poverty, the lower level of education of rural people, especially the poor, and the assumption that rural populations are less likely to observe principles of hygienic living. Furthermore, rural dwellers are regarded as less likely to obtain preventive immunizations, to have prenatal care during pregnancy, to eat a nutritionally balanced diet, and to obtain periodic health examinations for early disease detection. The poorest rural families, it is assumed, suffering discrimination on racial or ethnic grounds, exhibit fatalism and despondency so that medical attention is sought only when health problems become desperate (Roemer 1976:81).

This perspective on health problems in rural areas has been influential in shaping governmental policies toward rural health. Such a perception of rurality is supplemented by phrases such as: (1) " . . . many millions still face the handicaps of rural location and rural life" (Roemer 1976:v); (2) " . . . what other nations have attempted to do to overcome the obstacles of rurality" (Roemer 1976:v); (3) "the rural environment creates distinct obstacles that present low-income families with more difficulties within that environment" (Roemer 1976:68); (4) "In virtually all countries rural populations suffer health service disadvantages relative to urban populations" (Roemer 1976:108); and (5) "in summary, the total health families (volume of services in rural regions), while they have improved over the last quarter-century, are still somewhat lower in quantity than those serving large city populations, and their qualitative deficiencies are more serious" (Roemer 1976:79).

One obvious opposition throughout these judgements is the difference between rural and urban, with urban as the standard against which the quality of rural health is measured. It is assumed that "the best measure of the day-to-day medical care people receive is the rate of contact with physicians or dentists per person per year," with the standard being urban contacts (Roemer 1976:79). Thus, on the one hand, in urban areas higher quality of life means increased contact with physicians (assumed to mean better health care); while on the other hand, rural means lower quality life (poor education, health habits, and fatalism), thus lower quantity and quality of health care.

The paradigm produced by the above statements allows for the manipulation of symbols to create a reality that justifies the development of policies which serve the purposes of the medical profession and the needs of the government developing the policies. During the past few years, this model of rurality has crystalized and has prompted policy papers such as "Rural Health at the Crossroads" (Wartow 1979). In actuality, however, in the first part of this century, health statistics on cities indicate that urban areas were worse off than rural areas. It is also assumed that increased services are responsible for the distinctions having leveled out over the years since. Indeed, Roemer, reflecting this assumption, states that conditions of rural life reduce the risk of death from chronic diseases which primarily affect the aged, while they increase the risk of infections and traumatic conditions that are readily preventable with current medical knowledge. However, morbidity rates show that chronic illnesses are more a burden on rural peoples, particularly poor rural Blacks, than on urban people.

The suggested remedies to these perceived problems include: (1) increase resources both in personnel and facilities, (2) assure economic support for these services to all rural people and (3) maintain the quality of health service through social organization. These solutions can be facilitated through the principle of regionalization in which "small peripheral rural facilities come under the influence of large urban units" (Roemer 1976:116). Indeed, it is believed that deficiencies in health care will persist if rural health care depends solely on rural people. Thus, "rural health care can reach the level of urban health care only by tapping urban health" (Roemer 1976:117). Improvements cannot be expected within the boundaries of rural communities themselves. Rural people are too passive, uneducated, or unmotivated to take care of their needs as perceived by the health planners. Consequently, we find a steady broadening of the field of public responsibility for an individual's health. Indeed, it is suggested that "in the process of linking rural and urban resources, the government has had to play an increasing role" (especially government on the state and national level) and that the solution to "rural deficiencies in health resources and services will depend largely on deliberate social actions by the national government" (Roemer 1976:22).

Rurality and Policy

The development of a model for rurality (based on several metaphors) has recently culminated in policy papers and legislation specifically aimed at solving the problems of rural health. For example, a paper distributed in 1966 by the Department of Human Development Services (HEW) states that:

> For a number of years, federal decision makers have either ignored the health problems of rural areas or viewed them as insurmountable. Viewed against urban problems which were both more visible and thought to be more efficiently solvable, rural health has had a low priority, in terms both of the health agencies and those concerned with and involved in formulating rural development strategies. . . . The failure of past administrations in solving the crises of the cities has made rural areas more attractive both to settle in

and to improve. The success of a number of human service programs in rural areas, such as service integration and the rural health initiative, depends on policy-makers becoming aware of the need to address the major health concerns of nonmetropolitan areas (Wartow 1979).

In addition, we find that the Office of Rural Development reported in 1976 that one of the major barriers to the delivery of human services in rural areas is the lack of recognition on the part of bureaucrats, who predominantly live in large metropolitan areas, and that rural areas have unique problems that cannot be remedied with urban solutions. It is believed that there is little question that rural areas suffer from a number of severe resource deficiencies, in addition to geographic isolation and harsh climate; hence "alternatives to urban delivery models must be developed, tested, and implemented since the conditions of rural life require new and innovative solutions" (Wartow 1979:2). This new policy should place health care delivery within the framework of: (1) economic development that does not assume that economic opportunity and development must precede human resource development; (2) a cost-effective investment in health care that will improve the health status of rural people and thus enable them to become functioning, productive members of society; (3) expanded opportunities for employment in the health professions (the third largest sector of the U.S. economy) and (4) financial and organizational incentives to rural governments in service areas such as water, sewer, education, policy and fire protection.

This approach was supported by two policies that have made funds available for the development of health care in rural areas. They are: (1) the Health Underserved Rural Areas Program (HURA), established in 1974 for the purpose of conducting "research and demonstration projects for attracting physicians' assistants and nurse practitioners to rural scarcity areas to supplement and attract additional physicians manpower" (U.S. Senate 1974:88) and (2) the Rural Health Initiative (RHI), funded in 1975 to supplement start-up costs and initial operating deficits in communities which have succeeded in planning rural health care delivery projects. This initiative includes funding and support from the National Health Service Corps (Section 329 of Title III of the Public Health Service Act), Community Health Centers (Section 330 of Title III of the Public Health Service Act), Migrant Health Program (Section 319 of Title IV of the Public Health Service Act), Health Underserved Rural Areas Program (Section 1110 of Title XIX of the Social Security Act), and Appalachian Health Programs (Section 2020 of the Appalachian Regional Development Act).

These efforts, however, are not influencing the health status of rural areas as it was initially believed they would, and additional policies have been suggested that include: (1) the delegation of more power to the Office of Rural Health (legislative authority); (2) more comprehensive planning with other federal programs, especially the Hill-Burton Act and the Regional Medical Program; (3) more equitable distribution of Medicare and Medicaid in rural areas (less than 30% of Medicaid funds go to nonmetropolitan areas even though half the poor live in such areas); (4) additional facilities, medical personnel and transportation services and (5) more flexible funding. These policy recommendations are made in the spirit of the National Health Goal adopted by the Department of H.E.W. and the Department of Agriculture in 1977 whose purpose is:

> to promote the improvement of and equal access to quality comprehensive health care services (primary, preventive, and emergency medical services) for the population residing in all rural areas of the United States and its territories (HEW 1977).

To insure that this goal is implemented, Congress in 1980 enacted the Rural Development Policy Act, which states that the Secretary of Agriculture "shall conduct a systematic review of federal programs affecting rural areas to (A) determine whether such areas are benefitting from such programs in an equitable proportion to the benefits received by urban areas and (B) identify any factors that may restrict accessibility to such programs in rural areas or limit participation in such programs."

Key Metaphors for Action in Rural Areas: Evaluation and Values

An interpretation of the developmental processes of rural health policy must first look at the cause-and-effect sequence of the "rural problem" and its solutions. Obviously, the problem is located in the rural areas themselves and there is a danger of blaming the victim and fixing the cause with the area and with people that are not urban. This diverts attention to these areas and away from the social and political aspects of the larger problem, i.e., the broader structural context of American society. Rural peoples are thus separated out from the rest of society as requiring special policies and programs.

In the process of separating rural peoples out as a special problem, the key symbols of evaluation and subsequent action are used to measure the effectiveness of services. The symbolic gestalt for evaluation includes availability, accessibility and acceptability, cost, quality and continuity. As we have seen, these symbols are important in the overall health policy ideology that has provided the guidelines for changing the structure of the health system in the past few years. A guiding value in this model is that of equity; that is, the right of access to certain kinds of services, regardless of their maldistribution within the natural order. In other words, policies must be created to balance the distribution by changing the forces (social, economic, political) that brought about the maldistribution. Thus, a goal is set (political) and the system is forced to adapt to the changes brought about by the goal. Furthermore, the objectification of these systems is important within the framework of the overall cultural model that guides the policy process within this society. Consequently, certain facts are organized into a causal theory about health problems and then, based on the data base, appropriate intervention is recommended.

The data base that evaluates health status and health services is usually statistical. The majority of these data are gathered through the efforts of six federal surveys and inventories. They are: (1) basic vital statistics, (2) vital statistics followback surveys, (3) the National Health Interview Survey, (4) the National Health and Nutrition Examination Survey, (5) the National Hospital Discharge Survey and (6) the National Ambulatory Medical Care Survey (Gilford, et al., 1981). These statistics are broken down in a variety of ways, most often into the national, regional, state and county levels.

These data are analyzed to evaluate health status based on mortality and morbidity rates and health service based on variables such as availability, accessibility, cost and quality. The variables are operationalized in terms of standards set by the policy system through selecting research data on the optional ratios for the delivery of quality and quantity health care to the entire population. The standards and the ratios can change, mostly in response to social, economic and political phenomena and the changes in dominance of certain values and normative conceptions of health problems and their solutions. Realities shift as the political economy shifts, and vice versa. Consequently, the selection from the repertoire of data shifts and the cultural model of the policy process develops new causal theories; they then become generative metaphors (Schon 1979). Throughout this process, most health planners and policymakers make the assumption that health status is directly related to the availability and accessibility of medical care.

The Assumptions of Federal Evaluation Measures

In the past few years, the federal government has chosen to use two basic evaluation measures to identify rural areas with inadequate access to health care. They are Medically Underserved Areas (MUA), and the Critical Health Manpower Shortage Area (HMSA) (Figure 8). These measures make assumptions about health care utilization in rural areas which several recent studies have questioned (Kane, et al. 1978).

One of the most important components of federal programs aimed at alleviating geographic maldistribution of health resources is the identification and designation of the specific areas that are in need of health personnel. The earliest health personnel shortage areas designated were mandated by

	Medically Underserved Area (MUA)	Critical Health Manpower Shortage Area (CHMSA)	Health Manpower Shortage Area (HMSA)
Geographic unit	county, census tract or census division	county, group of census tracts or group of census divisions	designed area, population groups or facility
Basis of calculation	weighted combination of infant mortality rate, physician/pop'n ratio, % pop'n 65+, % pop'n below poverty level	<1 primary care MD per 4000 people (adjusted for contiguous areas)	<1 primary care MD per 3500 people or <1 per 3000 if specific indicators of need (adjusted for contiguous areas)
Programs affected	CHC, HURA, HMO. PL95-210	NHSC, HURA	NHSC, PL95-210
No. of areas designated	1967 (1977)	(1977) MD DDS 1106 854	(est. 1978) MD DDS 1300 950

Figure 8. Measures of Manpower Shortage Areas

1965 legislation providing for cancellation of repayment of the educational loans of health professionals if they served in shortage areas on the basis of specific ratios of several types of practitioners (physicians, dentists, nurses, pharmacists, veterinarians) to population. Special consideration was allowed for county or sub-county areas exhibiting an inaccessibility of medical services to the residents, a problem with the age or incapacity of practitioners, or a particular level of health problems.

In 1971, new criteria were established designating health shortage areas for the specialities physicians, optometrists and podiatrists. Most areas designated were entire counties, a result of data availability on that level. The physician shortage area list accounted for about 2/3 of all U.S. counties (Lee 1979; Gilford, et al. 1981).

There are several assumptions made about political boundaries and human behavior when designating counties as the key unit on which data are presented as arguments for shortage areas. First, in some states (most Western), rural areas are too large geographically to represent service areas and in other states (mostly Southeastern), the counties tend to be too small to be considered independent (Lee 1979). Second, the reliance on the physician-to-population ratio has a number of problems. According to Cordes (1976), these ratios (1) do not reflect possible differences in productivity among physicians and groups of physicians; (2) are too insensitive to quality considerations; (3) assume that populations are the same with respect to their needs for physician services and to the quantity of physician services demanded; (4) say little about the ease with which various groups may draw upon physician services; (5) assume that an area is a closed system—a reasonable assumption at the national level, but not with small geographic areas; and (6) do not consider the variations in the relationship among geographic size, continuous access and population density, factors related to the problems of accessibility and mobility. Another problem with this metaphor is that it does not consider nonphysician providers and may exaggerate the lack of personnel in some areas (Jagger 1978). Health personnel, other than medical doctors, may provide services to rural populations for most problems.

Another metaphor, that of the medically underserved area, began with the Health Maintenance Organization Act of 1973 that gave funding priorities to HMO's serving "medically underserved populations." Often the term "medically underserved area" is equated with rural areas. Indeed, a policy statement published by the National Rural Center states that "within the general category of rural, medically underserved areas are considered to have inadequate health care delivery services." Such areas tend to be sparsely populated and/or poor, sometimes with sizable minority populations. They tend to have higher-than-average infant mortality rates, more individuals over sixty-five than is average, and lower than average doctor-to-population ratios—all concerns of various kinds of medical care (Corman, et al. 1981).

In addition to physician/population ratios, the "medically underserved area" measure includes three indicators to designate underserved areas: (1) the infant mortality rate, an indicator of health status; (2) the percentage of population over the age of 65, an indicator of probable increased needs and demands for health care; and (3) the percentage of the population below the poverty level, an indicator of economic access barriers and increased needs for health care. As with health personnel shortage areas, county data are used as a basis for designating underserved areas.

The problem with this model is that it does not measure one single variable. Rather, it describes a relationship among population size, availability of services, socioeconomic characteristics of communities and health status. We do not know, however, how these variables may vary from area to area. Furthermore, the definition of this model can vary since the choice of these four variables is rather arbitrary (Wysong 1975). Another policy model created to designate health shortage areas was the Health Professions Education Assistance Act of 1976 (an effort to include more urban areas). The model includes the following features:

(1) Separate criteria are used for each type of health personnel.

(2) For each of these personnel types, there are three basic criteria:

(a) For designation of a geographic area, the area must be defined by approximate travel time to care.

(b) For most types of care, a modified population-to-practitioner ratio is still the basic indicator used. However, for those personnel types for which available data support such adjustments, either the population or the number of practitioners may be adjusted to reflect special needs or limitations, respectively.

(c) Personnel in a contiguous area must be considered; specifically, the travel time to reach them, whether they are already over used, and whether there are barriers (e.g., cultural) to their use.

(3) Particular population groups, such as Native Americans and migrants, may be designated as "shortage areas," even though the entire geographic area in which they reside does not qualify.

Inextricably related to the term "underserved" is the policy of increasing employment in the health professions and creating more jobs for the general public. In addition, we find that when combined with the general conception of rurality, these policies can be interpreted as an invitation for the invasion of urban-based agencies. The agencies, consequently, developed by policies such as the call for primary care clinics (which take on a momentum of their own) and community organization appear to be altruistic, but function to make rural peoples dependent on governmental programs and metropolitan areas. This process begins by defining a group as "deviant." They then become a target for special policies aimed toward making them conform to the urban norm (e.g., the 1980 Rural Development Act).

Furthermore, we find that political terms such as "a crisis" and "underserved" become symbolically meaningful in creating a frame (problem); they set a situation apart from others and create a need for special circumstances that require special attention in which sacrifices may be necessary for solving the problem. Edelman argues that "the reasons for almost all crises fall disproportionately on the poor, while the influential and the affluent often benefit from them" (1977:44). Thus, rural people have become a "problem"; they have become a homogeneous category (which tends to perpetuate stereotypes) toward which are aimed rather ambiguous policies which expand the service economy. Rural areas are becoming a market for service providers, a market which will snowball into the expansion of other businesses (drugs, for example). These processes indeed uphold the political economy of American society. Thus we are forced to ask the question, "Do these policies really create equal access to health care for all rural peoples or do the resources only service segments of the rural population which happen to fall into one of the measurements that have been culturally created in order to develop policy?" Who will those special programs benefit?

To answer these questions, it is important to track not only the meaning of these symbols within the cultural system but also the motivations and decision-making criteria in the minds of the decision makers. What are their causal models? Who do the solutions benefit? Obviously, they most benefit urban areas. The emphasis on regionalization and linkages with urban areas will function to expand the power base of the metropolitan medical facilities. The policies are unidirectional; resources and power flow from urban areas into rural areas (a new frontier). Policies that dictate a balance between rural and urban areas may appear on one hand to create an equity between the areas. On the other hand, however, they expand the power base of certain interest groups and individuals who may not adequately represent the interest of rural peoples. Interest group bargaining (pluralism) is believed to represent the democratic process in which the public interest is held to be adequately represented. What has been and what will be created by this process? Most probably it will create a network of planning that will provide more agencies and professional organizations (such as the newly created Association for Rural Development or the Rural Health Association) that in themselves become interest groups consisting largely of professionals who in turn will develop their own meanings and motivations, which will be reflected in their decision-making.

Metaphor and Reality

I suggest that the policies that have been constructed for rural areas are metaphors—socially constructed ideas of rural reality that are a mixture of "psychological assumptions, scientific concepts, value commitments, social aspirations, personal beliefs and administrative constraints" (Rein 1976:103). Furthermore, I suggest that this "reality" is a product of the processes involved in constructing a paradigm that takes on an objective quality which interest groups and/or policymakers assume as being concrete reality. In my opinion, this is done without much attention being paid to the social context and cultural meaning of the rural experience itself (Hill 1973). Indeed, "the less the knowledge base is empirically seen, the greater the influence of social and political factors in the interpretation and acceptance of data as knowledge" (Estes 1979:6). Berger and Luckman (1966) have extensively examined the social construction of reality and concluded that as definitions of reality become widely shared, they are institutionalized as part of the "collective stock of knowledge and although socially generated, such knowledge and expert opinion take on the character of objective reality regardless of inherent validity. Furthermore, it influences both the perception of the social problems and the solutions to these problems." Often, it seems that decision makers do not have feedback loops in their causal beliefs about social problems. That is, cognitively they do not have a general system of causal actions, but many causal beliefs which tend to contradict the feedback mechanism of social science models. Consequently, the motivations of individual decision makers become extremely important in analyzing their cultural system.

Decision makers' solutions have rarely considered the cultural and social context in which rural life exists and the meaning such a lifestyle has for an individual, family or community. One cultural system (health policy) does not connect with another cultural system (rural populations) in constructing health intervention strategies. Interventions could be created that incorporate the cultural experience of the people into the paradigm, e.g., how rural peoples differentially experience their environment and their health, and how rural peoples integrate the "problems" of rurality into their lives and explain them (not necessarily cope with them). Their bases for action could thus be strengthened and could render policies and actions more effective. Expanding the definition of rural reality may overcome the stigma that is being created by the current policy paradigm. The key question is "How can rural people gain access to our resource system without becoming a special interest group themselves, a group without power?"

The preceeding discussion of the perceptions of rurality and the policies that guide the health delivery system in rural areas illustrates the process involved in the creation of a rural paradigm. It is clear that these beliefs and attitudes about rural areas have affected the policies that have been developed in the past ten years and how they have been implemented in communities like Coberly. It is now time that we ask the following questions— Do these assumptions of reality impede rather than foster the quality of health care in rural areas? Can these policies solve the health care problems of rural people? And, lastly, does this developing rural paradigm uphold the existing power arrangements in our political and economic systems?

Linking Policy Metaphors to the State Level

With the establishment of federal health policies, their structures and ideology, the state level began to link into them through various organizational mechanisms. There is some disagreement about the nature and amount of federal influence on state health policy (Buntz, et al. 1978). Although the overall federal policies (their structure and ideology) are guidelines to state policies, a study by Buntz et al. (1978) concludes that in general, the political environment of a state tends to be a major factor determining the extent of federal influence. Two factors appear to be most important: state officials' knowedge of and participation in a program, and the degree to which the state accepts the program's basic goals. States were, until very recently, rather passive in their acceptance of federal programs and goals. It seems that change occurs only when the political environment of the state is receptive to change (Altensletter and Bjorkman 1975). Many states do not have a special office or agency for the planning of rural health. If attention is paid at all to rural health it is often done in a primary care section of state government which manages the major responsibility for the rural sectors of the population. Other sections, such as adult health or maternal and child care, also can plan for a state, although very often little, if any, attention is paid to the health problems in rural areas as opposed to urban areas. Furthermore, the Health Systems Agencies (the federal level) have in the past worked with rural areas to provide funding for primary health care clinics. Recently, however, their funding has been cut and, as a result, their effectiveness as a cooperating agency has decreased.

Using the general formula given on the federal level, states have established indicators for measuring the five service characteristics of availability, accessibility, cost, continuity and quality. For example, the State of Georgia uses: (1) manpower supply: availability and accessibility of primary health services; (2) Medically Underserved Areas: availability and accessibility of primary health services; (3) Primary Care Service Sites: availability and accessibility of primary health service and facilities, and (4) Third-Party

Payments and Coverage: accessibility and cost of primary care services (financial accessibility). Using these measures the health problems of the state emerge in terms of specific statistics, based on county data. From this data, specific policies for the state are formulated.

As of July, 1982, there were 85 geographical areas in Georgia designated by the federal government as having a shortage of primary care manpower. Included are 75 counties, some of them rural counties, and eight urban communities. The total population in these areas in 1980 was 1,449,000, or 28 percent of the total population of the state. Only 35 of these 85 areas have at least one federally financed health care provider (i.e., Rural Health Initiative, Urban Initiative, and Comprehensive Health Centers). In October, 1982, only 22 of these centers were receiving federal support, and five state funds. All of these centers are designed to provide services to low-income families as well as middle-class families (sliding scale payment basis). The target population for service by these 34 centers is 507,650 with only 7.8% having used them by August, 1982. The centers have been in operation from 26 months to one year, two thirds of them 2/3 staffed by National Health Services Corps assignees (MD, RN, Dentist).

Based on the national ratios, Georgia lags behind the availability and accessibility formulas for delivering health services. Its access physician supply is falling below the recommended percentages. In 1978 access physicians were 46 percent per 1000 people and in 1980 they were 45 percent (compared to the recommended 55 percent), while consultant physicians were 41 percent in 1978 and 43 percent in 1980, somewhat over the recommended 34 percent. This data led the State Health Planning and Development Agency to make the following statement:

> Shortages of primary care physicians coupled with the already demonstrated maldistribution of primary care physicians may be assumed to leave many [residents of the state] with greater access problems and with increased cost for obtaining needed primary care than would be the case if there were several (1982).

The structure of the public health care system, divided into the divisions of physical and mental health, has continued to function with a uniform policy, with problems handled on an individual basis and each county or regional area making its own implicit policies, depending on the individual leaders and their linkages to state agencies. It is the structure that has mattered and the structure that has adapted itself more or less to the community organizations. Within the past few years, however, the explicit ideology that has developed on the federal level, with its set of assumptions, beliefs and values, combined with specific sets of data, has filtered down to state levels and given health planners and policymakers symbols for change.

There is considerable debate on the "knowledge for what" question in the policy arena. Some authors feel that knowledge gained from research informs and shapes policy directions in both the private and public sectors (Weiss 1977). Others discuss the "two-communities" model (Caplan 1979). One faction feels that the goals of research and the goals of policy are so divergent that research has little influence on policy. On the other hand, others like Weiss (1977) believe that policy research does indeed influence decision-making but that in order to understand the contribution of social science to public policy, it is necessary to understand the processes of making public policy (Weiss 1979). Research which emphasizes problem solving or instrumental uses is evaluated by its direct contribution to decisionmaking rather than being evaluated on the basis of its general contribution to knowledge. The researchers who value the latter are accused of being indifferent to the policy arena and feeling that their research should be value-free. The researchers who value the former category are accused of conducting research in a less objective manner and thus are faced with the danger of "selling out to the system."

Research and Policy: Which Guides Which?

Whichever values the social science researchers in health services adhere to, their research has had a minimum impact on the formation of policy (Bice, 1981). The blame has been laid primarily "on the researchers and their styles and communication" (Eichhorn and Bice 1973). The harshest critics feel that "social science research is irrelevant to policymakers . . . [or] it is simply not packaged in ways that policymakers can comprehend, or disseminated through channels that reach their attention" (Bice 1981:5). The literature is replete with studies that show what kinds of research are more useful than others or what characteristics are more important than others in presenting data (Lingwood 1979; Weiss-Bucuvalas 1977; Caplan 1975; Lehman & Waters 1979). Many of these studies contradict one another. So the question may be "What kind of research influences policy?"

Research on health issues which is grounded in the theoretical and methodological approaches of social science frames its questions within its general paradigm. Policy uses such knowledge within its own frame or ideology to make choices. These two frames, when combined, produce policy analysis and policymaking. The processes of interaction of these two frames are interesting in that the dominant metaphors of the policymakers guide the research questions and consequently the answers. They allow the unfamiliar to become familiar by using experience to interpret the data via analogy and to identify the cause of the problem. The analogy also dictates a logical solution within the boundaries of the frame.

While research tends less to guide policy (although it is indeed useful in the policy process), Weiss (1979) found that the need for information and the ways in which this need is met within the policy arena depend upon the contexts surrounding the formation and implementation of policy. He identified these contexts as (1) the content of policy issues; (2) the degree to which decision-making is centralized; and (3) the characteristics of the individuals and organizations that implement policy. The contexts are, in reality, defined by the dominant metaphors or ideologies of the policymakers in power. They frame the parameters of policy and delineate the areas of relevant research. Indeed, Anderson (1966) found that public consensus tends to create frameworks within which research priorities are set. So the social scientists who feel they are conducting value-free research are really providing additional knowledge to uphold a particular ideology. What else sets the boundaries of research? Thus, social scientists are part of the political process itself.

Facts Versus Values

"Public policy inherently mixes facts and values" (Bice 1981) in very complicated webs which are nearly impossible to untangle. This complex structure becomes clear when the stories that produce problem-setting frames are examined. A problem is delineated through the use of the metaphors which policymakers believe to be true. The basis for setting problems is a combination of fact and interpretation of fact. Recently Hanft (1981) has pointed out that social science data must be reliable in order to determine the needs of a population and assess the consequences of intervention and further, that the most basic social data bases are the census and vital statistics. Given all the problems involved in collecting census information, the policy problem involved is how to organize the data according to a cause-and-effect model.

To illustrate the problem, Hanft discusses the problem of "assumptions" in the debate between proponents of market competition and proponents of governmental regulation in health service. She states:

> There is a major political debate about the factors that cause health care inflation and the methods that might control escalating costs. The health care industry is complex and composed of many interrelated parts. It is a service industry that, unlike other service industries, faces choices related to life, death and disability. The good produced is not merely an economic good, but also involves fundamental issues of social justice. Yet most attention is paid to the economic issues: debates on access to care, content of health services, and forms of delivery of services are cast in economic terms. The two poles of opinion in the economic debate are the competition school and the regulation school (1981:599-600).

The two opposing forces make several rather opposing assumptions or, to put it another way, the frames are bounded by the metaphors they have used to set their perceptions of the key health problems and their solutions. The "free market" or "competitions" approach assumes:

(1) A free market approach will work in health care;
(2) Consumers have enough information to make rational choices;
(3) Suppliers have free entry into the economic market;
(4) Most demand is created by consumers, and demand can be withheld or delayed;
(5) Demand induced by providers can be reduced through economic incentives;
(6) Prices will fall if demand falls or supply increases;
(7) If consumers directly pay for services (rather than through third party payers) they will act as rational purchasers—shopping for the best buy;
(8) Supply will expand or contract in relation to demand.

On the other hand, the "regulation school" makes the following assumptions:

(1) A free market approach will not work in health care;
(2) Consumers can never have sufficient technical information to make truly informed choices; there is not free entry of suppliers into the economic market because of licensure and other constraints related to quality;
(3) The life, death and disability results of choice, combined with the need for highly technical information, require that the consumer have an agent represent him—the physician;
(4) Demand is often created by the agent who has an economic stake in providing services;
(5) Direct payment at time of use may influence demand marginally, but it has less than normal influence when the product is related to urgent health needs or pain;
(6) Direct payment at time of use acts as a barrier to access for some groups, particularly low-income groups (Hanft 1981:600-601).

Ironically, there is very little empirical data that conclusively supports one position or another and in what there is, neither approach is entirely supported (Hanft 1981), although this debate is a relatively old one. Could there be benefits in not collecting the appropriate data, which would continue to make the situation ambiguous at best? Ambiguity does serve an important function in mediating contradictory models of health reality.

Hence, the data continues to be "inadequate" so both views of reality can continue to function in the political system and, at the same time, continue to "need" further research. The goals are contradictory and the continuation of one approach is necessary to the continuation of the other and seems to be essential for compromise at any one point.

Furthermore, the political process, with its opposing metaphors, continues to infer cause from interpreted effects (health problems) using social science research. Hanft feels, however, that the problems of using research data in policy analysis and policymaking lie not in the political process's interference with the use of data, but "in the use of different data sources, the objectivity and validity of the data, and the differences in perspectives or the disciplinary school of the analyst or the political philosophy of the policymaker" (Hanft 1981:608-609). In this statement, Hanft has pointed out the key processes involved in the perpetuation of opposing frames. The selection of data, the analysis of data, the interpretation of data and the application of data all depend on what questions are asked, what segments of reality are chosen for study, and what paradigm guides the interpretation of the significant factors to explain the research problem. Again, Hanft feels that "the public must also become aware that most decisions made are based on the interaction of political and social values with data" (1981:612).

Fact, Value, and Policy

The "fact-value" dilemma has been discussed by a variety of scholars, the most lucid ideas, in my opinion, being those of Rein (1976). He feels that policy analysis can be viewed as an interpretation of beliefs. He states that "the crucial issues in a policy debate are not so much matters of fact as questions of interpretation. Theories of why things are as they are prove to be difficult to document and to refute. The lines of causality can often be reversed with equal plausibility, and there is not an easy way to choose among the conflicting interpretations which follow" (1976:12). Indeed, "social phenomena cannot be understood in isolation from the framework of thought which organizes evidence, interprets it and infers policy decisions which are consistent with it. A better appreciation of these frameworks or ideologies is crucial to understanding how social science and policy influence each other" (1976:15). As knowledge is expanded through research, it is used selectively to justify actions reached through the policy process.

According to Rein, research "provides factual information, that is empirical evidence in the form of quantitative estimates and/or qualitative experiences which can be organized to relate the values we hold, and to confirm or repudiate our beliefs about the functioning of society, institutions and people" (1976:38). He cleverly demonstrates his ideas by discussing opposing frameworks of thought about the relationship between poverty and ill health.

Three different frames are found in the literature that link these two variables—research allocation, personal and social theory and institutional performance. Rein feels that the findings of empirical research cannot be isolated from the theoretical and policy perspectives that guide the research. Each frame leads to very different priorities for action, although the literature fails to directly confront the conflict among the different paradigms. This becomes clear when causal links are analyzed. The question becomes, is poverty the cause of ill health or is it the consequence of ill health? Rein demonstrates how the opposing frames use social science research to conclude that both these theories are correct depending on which assumptions the researcher used in the research. The policies prescribed to restructure the situation obviously depend on which research the policymaker chooses to utilize as evidence of his/her perspective. Rein concludes his arguments by stating that "we must accept the position that objective evidence does not permit us to choose among competing ideologies or frameworks of thought" (1976:252) and that multi-paradigmatic research must be supported in social science.

This discussion is meant not to imply that the basis for decision-making on the part of policymakers does not change. Paradigms change and people's ideas change over time. Although a synchronic view can help us understand the processes of symbolic decision making, from a diachronic perspective, values and ideology adjust to the stresses and strains of social and cultural change. According to the findings of Weiss and Bucuvalas (1977) federal decision-makers are receptive to research that does not support their ideas. It makes them rethink their assumptions, although it is unclear how such controversial research affects their decision making. Likewise, Knorr (1977) reports that social science data is both symbolic and instrumental among decision-makers in Austria, although the utilization of the data is indirect and difficult to trace through the decision-making process.

In the previous section I examined the key metaphors used in defining the health problems in rural areas and the proposed solutions to these problems. Both the problems and the solutions are based on selecting research data to uphold the basic assumptions of the varying paradigms, both in the social sciences and in the policy arena, and from a cultural system that provides meaning to both policymakers and social scientists.

8

The Convergence and Divergence of People and Policy

It is the political task of the social scientist—as of any liberal educator— continually to translate personal troubles into public issues, and public issues into the terms of their human meaning for a variety of individuals. It is his task to display in terms of his work—and, as an educator in his life as well—this kind of sociological imagination (C. Wright Mills 1963:187).

This book has explored the complex cultural and social issues involved in linking the health systems of groups of people in a community to rural health policy. This study was designed to examine the categorical differences among groups in a community rather than to extensively describe one group, in order to provide a better understanding of the various groups' differential linkages to the health system. Analyzing the Coberly community in terms of its categorical structures is a necessary step in order to make valid statements about the variation in health behavior and beliefs, illness response, and differential linkages to health services. As I discussed in previous chapters, these linkages are to individuals and groups on the community, regional, state, and national levels of the health system.

Processes of mediation (linkages) between all levels involved in macrolevel and microlevel studies are "unequal and contradictory" (Wolf 1982; Mintz 1977, Silverman 1979 & Trouillot 1984). Inequality refers to power relations while contradictions refer mainly to the divergent of the cultural models of people and policymakers. Dewalt and Pelto (1985) state that " . . . we have few theoretical and methodological guidelines for articulating the linkages between microlevels and macrolevels," and this problem is among the most vexing issues in social science research (1985:1). The data collected for this book was an attempt to reconstruct the "scenes of activities" that brought about changes in health services to Coberly. Connecting these events and the cultural models that guide health policies with the observed and reconstructed health behavior and cultural models of the groups in Coberly has led me to conclude that it is crucial to discover the convergent and divergent processes of behavioral and cultural models on all the levels of mediation.

This approach has both theoretical and practical applications to the study of rural health. Ortner (1984) feels that theory in anthropology in the 1980s is attempting to understand how society and culture are produced, reproduced and transformed through human intention and action. Emphasis is placed on action, the decision-making of individuals in a community within the larger sociopolitical context, in order to understand and explain the interaction between individuals/groups and "the system." We have seen in Coberly that this is not a one-way process—people who are not involved in the policy process make decisions about their health behavior which often contradict the cultural models of "the health system." We get, then, a clearer understanding of how and why health culture is produced, reproduced and transformed. In this process, the health system is, at the same time, a system of social relations, economic arrangements, political processes, cultural categories, norms and values and emotional patterns— all components that integrate into the health order and action system.

On the practical side, factors pertaining to the way people and policies converge or diverge are important for constructing culturally and socially appropriate policies for the delivery of health care services. Changes in policy come from "the system," but how the people cooperate or accept the changes depends on how much the cultural models of the policy makers and those of the people overlap. The failure of primary health care in Coberly illustrates the importance of understanding the cultural system of people on the macrolevel and how it gets produced or reproduced on the local level. "The system" may "blame the victim," i.e., without adequate attention paid to how a transformation is mediated (as in the establishment of the PHC clinic), which makes it easy to blame the people of Coberly, for example, rather than the health system for its failure. Many of the health problems of Coberly could be planned for and treated more effectively with a knowledge of the ways in which the social and cultural models of the health policy process and the people converged and diverged in their production, reproduction, and transformation.

Convergent Processes

The major issues on which the people of Coberly agree ideologically and behaviorally with the current health policies involve the medicalization process and the production of knowledge by the medical system. Such convergences in cultural models and behavior can be explained by two factors: 1) unequal power relations and 2) the production of meaning by the political and corporate aspects of medicine. Everyone involved in the mediation process participates in the same society and, for the most part, in the same health system. As we have seen, however, their cultural models are not homologous and the motivations for their behavior diverge and converge depending on their socioeconomic levels and, consequently, on the power differentials among the levels in the system.

In the past decade, much has been said about the medicalization of American society. An extreme perspective on this process has been put forth by Illich (1975), who feels that the medical establishment has become a threat to health through social, clinical, and structural iatrogenies. Although the validity of his argument is debatable, he does bring to our attention the fact that an increasing number of behaviors have been incorporated into the model of disease and illness. Maladies that were once considered to be the responsibility of the criminal justice system have now switched systems and have joined the medical system. Sedgwick has proclaimed that "the future belongs to illness" because "we are going to get more and more diseases, since our expectations of health are going to become more expansive and sophisticated" (1973:37). The medicalization of society has socialized people into increasingly utilizing the medical system for illness episodes that could be dealt with just as easily through alternative health resources. Going to a doctor and getting a shot or pills has become a metaphor for wellness. Many of the people of Coberly believe that these are the best alternatives for getting well, a belief that has become a cultural value in our society. Obtaining more medical services, however, does not necessarily mean better health.

Although policymakers and the medical corporate structure believe that medicalization is a positive step toward better health, there are those who are concerned about the overmedicalization of American society. For example, Carlson states:

> Today, few patients have the confidence to care for themselves. The inexorable professionalization of medicine, together with reverence for the scientific method, have invested practitioners with sacrosanct powers, and correspondingly vitiated the responsibility for the rest of us for health (1975:141).

This has resulted in a dominance of the medical profession in planning health services and structures and a loss of the ability of some groups of people to believe they can take care of themselves. While the people of Coberly generally do not give up their sense of power to a doctor, many revere the ideology of scientific medicine and extend their expanded health behaviors into the paradigm. Carlson's statements do apply, moreover, to the increasing dependence on the medical system which has caused them to lose or give up (no longer transmit to younger generations) the resources they have traditionally had with which to help themselves. Carlson, however, predicts an end of medicine which "is not the end of health but the beginning" (1975:231) since medical care has affected health less than is generally assumed. Of course this is because social and environmental factors are affecting health status more substantially than are viruses.

The boundaries of health care, then, are expanding and extend beyond the biomedical model traditionally used for setting health policies. On the local level, some people are aware of social and environmental factors which affect health but not all. This transition is beginning to happen in Coberly mainly among middle and upper income groups. The "health consciousness" of the late 1970's and 1980's has increased their knowledge of healthy ways to live and some are taking their health into their own hands and using alternatives beyond biomedicine. Through their increasing awareness of the complex factors that influence health, all groups can become empowered to actively transform the kinds of health knowledge that are produced and reproduced in the community. This process will cause contradictions (divergences) in the cultural models of the mediators of the health system that will eventually affect policies so that they will become more convergent with people's beliefs and behaviors.

Both those on the political/institutional level and the people on the local level believe overall that modern scientific medicine is the best kind of treatment. With the expansion of public health and medical services to the rural areas of Georgia in the middle part of this century came an alternative system of explanation for illness and treatment. Medical services became increasingly an option for the people of Coberly. The option was weighted however; it came from the dominant power group in the society, and along with it came the production of new health knowledge that ultimately created a transformation in the cultural models of the people. This transformation, however, was not uniform: some groups bought into the dominant medical system more than did others. The impact of the medicalization process on people depends upon the structural position and cultural models of the impacted group.

Another process of convergence, inextricably bound to medicalization, is the production and distribution of medical knowledge by the medical system which encompasses a complex of symbols and meanings that dominate a major part of the beliefs and behaviors of the groups in Coberly. The irony of such convergence is that the areas of overlapping meaning between folk models and medical models of diagnosis and treatment (science and technology) are not the areas that can effectively treat a large number of the health problems of the people of Coberly—a point that cannot be overemphasized in linking policies and people. This was demonstrated in Chapters 6 and 7.

People gain medical knowledge from their family and community, their contacts with the health system, and from the media. Health personnel participate, for the most part, in the beliefs and expected behavior of the system they represent. They also must behaviorally adhere to the current health policies of the society—whatever the policy "frames" or "problem-setting" priorities are in a given political administration (payment procedures, eligibility requirements, types of services rendered, etc.). This health cultural system and the particular policies that affect the delivery of rural health services produce and reproduce knowledge for the people.

Studies over the past decade or so conclude that the media ("media medicine") have a major impact on the health knowledge and behavior of people. Specific groups are, however, selective in what kind of information gets translated into behavior. In large measure, the selecting process is guided by socioeconomic levels, as demonstrated in Chapters 4 and 5. People who can afford alternative healing modalities such as chiropractors, exercise classes, "health foods" and the like are more influenced by the information in the media on these areas, while lower income peoples are more influenced by information about over-the-counter medicines that are deemed helpful for their health problems. Corporate advertisers also seek to transform health behavior by creating new meanings about causes and treatment of health problems. The institutions in American society that shape cultural models are powerful forces and should be looked at more closely. Suffice it to say here that medical institutions (including corporations) are out to make a profit, and by shaping the cultural models of the health personnel who link to the people and directly shaping those of the people through the media, are crucial factors in explaining the convergence—in terms of ideology and behavior—of policy and people.

A critical assessment of a health system and the congruencies among its parts involves analyzing the levels of political and economic power and the actual benefits (and beneficiaries) of specific policies and planning strategies, as well as assessing illness and health patterns of the people in a community. The uncoordinated changes in health policy in the U.S. over the past two decades have failed to bring about changes in the health order that would equalize and provide care to all citizens of the U.S. Such a goal would involve a change in the social order as well as a change in the ideology of the power brokers who make and implement policies that will eventually legitimate the changes in a society. Navarro (1975) has documented the fact that corporate and upper-middle class persons have considerable influence on the policy-making bodies of American health institutions. He argues that control over these institutions mirrors the pattern of class dominance in other areas of the political and economic systems. Alford (1975) similarly found that there is a high probability that health elites will take a public position consistent with the interests of their specific organizations. Health policies uphold the existing dominant structure and culture in American society and consequently, converge with part of the structure and culture of people.

Divergent Processes

As with convergent processes, the factors that create incongruent cultural models and behavior can be traced to inequality in the social system, as reflected in the ineffectiveness of health policies, the differential health models among the people of Coberly and the people who make and implement policies, and the mismatching of medical services with peoples' needs. Rural people generally pay more for health care than do urban people. I did not find, however, that physical access is a problem for most people of Coberly. Differential knowledge, ineffectual health promotion and education, and belief in alternative pathways to the treatment of illness appear to be the major reasons for groups of people in Coberly to link differently to the health system. I hasten to say that the very poor and pregnant women do have access problems, and, as a consequence, they are either not treated or have babies who die in infancy, as discussed in Chapter 4.

The divergent process that most affects the health of the people of Coberly is the failure of rural health care policies to address the major health problems of the people. The changes in disease patterns in the U.S. from acute to chronic disorders have disproportionately affected people who live in rural areas (Frate, Johnson, and Sharpe 1985). Their problems call for preventive solutions, which an active primary health care program could provide. The major health problems of Coberly cannot be attributed solely to biological causes, nor can individuals (in terms of behavior or emotion) be held totally responsible for their own health status. Likewise, the environmental, social, and cultural components of health contribute to, but are not the only cause of, health problems or wellness. I agree with Elling (1978), who argues that the most important cluster of variables affecting health status are the distribution of wealth, the level of education, sanitation, housing conditions, and patterns of life of a population. Consequently, "the problem of disease is largely resident in the society" (1978:110). Indeed, under capitalism, "there is often a contradiction between the pursuit of health and the pursuit of profit" (Doyal 1981). Incremental policy changes on the macrolevel have only sporadically improved health services to rural people and as discussed in Chapters 6 and 7, only address issues within the dominant medical cultural model. Indeed, many rural legislative changes reach only a few segments of the population and many of them are advantageous in furthering the bureaucratic structure of the health system. Changes of this kind are not systematic and tend to work in a haphazard fashion, which partially explains the failure of health promotional and educational programs within the primary health approach.

Another process of divergence involves the differential cultural models of the people who participate in the health system. Chapter 4 and 5 explored the models of the people and how they all actualized, while Chapter 7 discussed the models in the institutional settings that create and implement policy. The people in the community are only vaguely aware of the motivations and objectives of the dominant system. While some of the objectives change with different governmental administrations, who have different "frames," the system on the local level generally is reproduced without transformations that impact the health status of the people.

I discovered a discrepancy between two points of view regarding the health needs of the community: that of the health planners who instigated the clinic and that of the targeted population. However, the discrepancy is not one that would have been easily predicted. Thirty-five percent of the people of Coberly said a doctor was the biggest health care need of the area. Twenty-one percent of those qualified their answers with phrases such as "a good doctor," "a good one that's concerned about everybody," "a doctor besides the health center," "a doctor . . . so they wouldn't have to drive," and "people in this area aren't sick that much." Only one person said a health care clinic was the biggest health care need. Forty-six percent of the interviewees listed services provided by the primary health care clinic as meeting the health care needs of the county.

These ambivalent feelings about the clinic and its services became a focus of our probing. One reason for these feelings is the expectation of having a doctor in the town for the health order to be complete. Coberly had a doctor for many years. Then, for an interval of ten years, people had to go outside the county. Many of the people who said a doctor was a need in the area feel that "the town" needs a doctor because it is without what it had before, but that they as individuals do not need a doctor in town. Thus the town, an entity in itself, has an unfulfilled need.

People also want the security of a doctor close at hand in case of emergencies, and they want the doctor to be a part of the town. Several respondents plan to continue to see their established doctors for routine visits or minor emergencies that are not acute. Of course, the primary health care clinic was established to handle routine family health care, and record transfers from former doctors are required of patients. The clinic does not handle emergencies. So we find another discrepancy between the patients' and the health planners' perceptions of health needs.

The health cultural models of the groups of people in Coberly, while convergent regarding acceptance of and belief in the efficaciousness of scientific medicine, are incongruent regarding the causes and treatments of illnesses, the cost and expectations of the dominant system. Not only did I find incongruences between the system and the people of Coberly but also among the different social classes in Coberly. All groups, however, use health modalities other than the medical system—their health behavior goes beyond the medical system—demonstrating that they are active participants constituting culture and transforming it, while at the same time they are constituted by the culture of the medical system. People in all groups transform and reproduce models for health that guide their health behavior. The variations among the models can be explained by the differences between their experiences in linking to the health care system. The basis for the differential linkages is their status in the social structure. All are active decision-makers who use the knowledge they have, integrate additional information into their cultural models and thus create divergent health models and behavior.

Linking People and Policy

Since the cultural models of the hierarchy of groups involved in making health policy and the delivery of health services on the one hand, and the utilization of health services, on the other hand, both converge and diverge, culturally and socially appropriate ways to link them together must consider the similarities and the differences. Linking people into the policy process and linking the process into people involves, ideally, fostering communication and understanding between the groups involved. It is not that simple, however. Such a solution ignores power within the system and the direction in which power flows—policy level to people level. While people are not passive recipients of the dictates of dominant groups, their alternative choices for action are bounded by the system (culture and structure) in which they are acting; hegemony is, however, never total. Consequently, changes can be made in at least two directions. The groups on the receiving end of policy decisions can decide to live within the boundaries of the decisions and adjust their behavior and cultural models accordingly. New options will be given to people over time and they can either accept or reject them. A second direction involves people taking more of an active role in policy formulation and implementation. Such change would demand a shift in the existing culture and structure of all groups involved in the health order.

It would require a "redesign rather than a shakeup" (Newell 1975) on both the policy level and the people level.

The second direction is a kind of health praxis in which the links between the health circumstances of rural people and the actions needed to change those circumstances can be realized through democratic action. Such a strategy is grounded in the ability of people to reflect upon their human health condition and to take actions that will change that condition, if change is necessary. It also assumes that the people who make health policies will recognize and act upon "frames" that are generated by the people. Praxis is a dialectic between criticism and activity which joins theory to practice. It is a disciplined uniting of thought and practice (Gramsci 1971) through providing guidelines for practice—changes deemed necessary in the health system—since practice without theory is haphazard and ineffective to segments of a population within a region/community.

The obvious question at this point is "Which people?" Who participates in a rational praxis approach to linking policies and people? Which groups of people who live in the community or specific people in the health systems? A Marxist would suggest that the lower income peoples of Coberly are oppressed and that the ruling class has successfully persuaded the lower classes to accept its own moral, political and cultural values (Gramsci 1971). The social order of health imposed by outside forces is, for the most part, accepted by the people of Coberly as a crucial health alternative. It is appreciated rather than being thought of as a crumb thrown to them by a ruling class. Rational health praxis is foreign to the people of Coberly and changes in the health order through revolutionary means would certainly be rejected. Such a praxis would, however, involve people on all levels of the health hierarchy and importantly, would take the social and cultural systems of both the policy makers and the people into consideration.

The lower income peoples of Coberly are indeed receiving less quality health care, pay more for it, and have fewer options. This is not just because of economics, but also because of their powerless position in the health structure. While economic factors are important in explaining the overall health status and behavior of Coberly's citizens—factors such as lack of money to purchase enough and/or nutritious foods or to obtain proper prenatal and postnatal care—ideological ones related to beliefs about the causation and treatment of illnesses also contribute to the health behavior and status of the people. Data collected in this study indicate that there are fundamental differences between the social classes and ethnic groups of Coberly. There is no "community health perspective." So, we are back to the same question: Who should represent the community in a rational approach to praxis? My answer is that all classes and ethnic groups and their ideologies should be represented; however, the idea of applying the democratic process to health policy in this way contradicts the current practice of decision-making based on a capitalistic economy. Indeed, the ideal of guaranteed equity in health care fundamentally contradicts the current policy "frames" or cultural models of the power structure that makes health policy in American society.

Linkage Problems

The problems of delivery of health services for Coberly are related to the various meanings of illness episodes, illness responses, access, and utilization. As we have seen, rural health policies that have been developed in the past decade have placed emphasis on providing greater access to health care facilities. However, the term "access" has a different meaning to health planners and policymakers than to the people themselves. Furthermore, these varied meanings are linked to the utilization of health facilities. Access is not a unidirectional process. As we have seen, policy makers view access in terms of the distances one has to travel to a clinic or hospital and the doctor/patient ratio. The assumption is that if health facilities are close enough to people and doctors are available, then people will utilize the health services. Underutilization and overutilization are then policy terms that are translated into numbers depending on a rather arbitrary set of criteria.

When one analyzes such terms from the people's perspective, however, as I did with the data from Coberly, they have meanings which in many respects are the antithesis of their meanings from a policy perspective. Access, for example, includes not only physical access but is also a social and cultural process, thus can also be viewed in terms of the scientific medical system's having access to the patients. Therefore, access needs to be measured not just in terms of distance or doctor/patient ratio but also in terms of communicating or intervening on a social and cultural level; i.e., building linkages to people's health systems. We could ask, "Does a clinic have access to the patients?" If not, the reasons for its underutilization are extended beyond cost or transportation problems into the realm of social and cultural systems. The decision-making process on the part of people is based as much on these variables as on material ones. Consequently, definitions of utilization and needs and how they are to be implemented in practical terms—i.e., decisions about health care—are multidimensional, a fact which is generally not reflected in health policies.

"Access" to a medical facility in Coberly does not guarantee its utilization. Over 70 percent of Coberlians indicated they would not go to the newly established clinic or would go only for emergency care, and 84 percent of these do not have problems with transportation to medical facilities. This attitude on the part of the people who were targeted as the recipients of the clinic's services was surprising at first, but made sense as we began to analyze the data. Eighty percent of the interviewees were utilizing medical facilities in other counties and expressed a reluctance to change. Building linkages to people involves more than just building a new structure and staffing it.

A major problem for health planners then, is that of access and utilization as meaningful concepts and the different ways these concepts are interpreted by providers and consumers of health care. Lack of access to medical facilities in rural areas is often cited as a major obstacle to reasonable health care for the areas' residents. Scant economic resources, geographic isolation and transportation problems are some of the factors that limit access to health care. Policymakers and planners have operated under the assumption that by removing some or all of these obstacles, they can provide better health care. This assumption neglects factors such as trust and perceived mutual understanding between patient and provider, belief in the provider as able to help or cure specific conditions, and perhaps most importantly, the willingness of the provider to share the responsibility for decisions concerning health or illness through discussion of problems and information exchanges. In other words, the people want to be treated as individuals who know their own normal health levels, and who can take responsible actions when understandable explanations about their health or illness status are given them.

It appears, then, that access and needs must be understood as operating in two directions. Not only does access have to be provided for targeted rural populations, but access to the people by the facility has to be taken into consideration. These statements should not be interpreted as a "blame the victim" attitude. Most of the people we talked to demonstrated their unwillingness to place themselves in a victim role either by their health attitudes or their behaviors. Most are as interested in prevention as they are cures. But utilization of medical facilities depends on intangible factors that should be taken into consideration in expanding the medical care system. Thacker, et al. (1979) came to similar conclusions in their study in rural North Carolina. The removal of legal and financial barriers to primary health care made little impact on the patterns of health care delivery established before changes such as mandatory integration of health services and the availability of government financing programs. Neither of these changes, thus, ensured utilization of medical services according to need, nor guaranteed equal access to care.

Changing Policies and People

One of the major points of this book is that health care is an issue that goes beyond the medical model. Health is a societal concern and major changes in health policies change the social order—the policies affect the everyday lives of people in the various communities throughout a society. As demonstrated in Chapter 7, priorities for policies are based on the cultural system of the policymakers (based on the fit between the ideology and the political economy) and not on the cultural system of the people (Chapters 4, 5, 6). Changing policy and people is a challenge to the entire social system if all levels are to be allowed to participate in setting policy. The major health policy issues that have emerged in the past decade, according to Crichton (1981:251) are:

(1) How can health policy contribute to a better social order?

(2) What impersonal or general programs of service should be developed as a matter of right through regulation and redistribution for groups in a particular society needing health care and for at-risk groups needing particular help . . . ?

(3) To what extent can personalized services by health professionals continue to be delivered as a matter of professional caring and as a matter of individual justice?

(4) What relationship should public programmers have with the existing privately developed institutions, programmers and personnel in the system of care?

(5) How can individual consumers be made more self-reliant, less dependent on medical services for all kinds of counseling?

(6) How best can prerogatives or rights be distributed among health service providers?

A reframing of policies on the creation of new "stories"—metaphors for change—is in order if we are truly concerned with improving people's health statuses. If, indeed, society regards health as an end, "the nation must take steps to consider its health promotion and illness prevention policies and its environmental conservation and development policies" (Crichton 1981:253). As an issue of society, policymakers must reframe the problems and their solutions that integrate the goals of the society with those of the individual. Again, Crichton states that "when individuals regard health as an end, they do pay attention to life style," but if they regard health as a means, "they may not choose a healthy lifestyle if it conflicts with their chosen pattern of daily living" (1981:253). The data from Coberly substantiates these statements and indicates that changes of lifestyle must occur within a participatory framework among the heterogenous groups on the local level. This requires, however, changes on all levels of society and culture.

Alford (1979) argues that the health system is remarkably resistant to change (dynamics without change) due to a struggle between different major interest groups operating within the context of a market society. These groups include the professional monopolies that control the major health resources, the corporate rationalizers, and the community populations. Although this pluralistic model is currently regarded as the most equitable approach to policymaking, Alford feels that change is not likely to occur in the health system unless the legitimacy of pluralism is rejected. He states that "given a system which cannot provide decent care for all because of the domination by the private sector and thus a continuing 'crisis,' there is increasing pressure upon government to step in . . . because of the dominance of the private sector, government cannot act in a way which could change the system without altering the basic principles of private control over the major resources of the society" (1975:343).

Rational rural health policies can clarify the present contradictions between the inability of the private sector to provide adequate and equal health care, the impossibility of the public sector's compensating for the inadequacies of the private sector, and the expectations and needs of the people. The alternative policies suggested shift policy making and planning toward a participatory model rather than a pluralistic one (Hill 1986). I am not making the mistake of equating policy and action as synonymous which Sher (1983) warns against. A systems approach to change assumes actions to change the health order, not just to change policies. Sher states that:

> the political invisibility of rural constituencies—at least on non-agricultural issues—has meant that uniquely rural concerns routinely rank at the bottom among governmental priorities. Since public policy cannot pay equal attention to all possible issues at the same time, and since governments are prone to allowing a continuous stream of "crises" to dictate the public agenda, those elements of society—like "marginal" rural population—that tend to be politically passive, poorly organized or simply out of the sight of policy makers tend to be the recipients of benign neglect and selective inattention by the government (1983:10).

In the past decade, we find that the health care system has not suffered from underexposure. The amount of information amassed, however, contributes little towards the resolution of policy questions because the policy problem is not due to insufficient information or faulty analysis, but rather an inability to resolve conflicting and competing interests among powerful actors (Mechanic 1981; Alford 1975). Indeed, Mechanic says that with the current emphasis on cost containment, it is difficult to promote the interests of some groups without taking resources or other advantages from those who already have them, and this establishes considerable tension in the policy-making arena. I have analyzed these competing interests within the framework of the symbols that give meaning to the policy arena—symbols that often are in conflict with the symbolic logic of the people. It is also important to understand the politics of health within the context of capitalism, a system that fosters class differences, which, as we have seen, make for differences in health status, health knowledge, and access to health services. An understanding of this relationship between health, illness and capitalism is necessary in order to bring about changes in the health order to provide health for all (Doyal 1981).

Summary

The key issues involved in this study are the conflicts between homogeneity and heterogeneity, class and inequality in a community and society, and how these issues influence or can influence the delivery of health care services. In my analysis, class factors override other variables in explaining health behavior and beliefs and, as we found, the ideology of health policies and planning is more in harmony with that of upper income peoples. Lower income peoples are not fatalistic or disorganized. They want to become involved in the curative and preventive aspects of their health. Although the metaphors that frame these groups' health realities differ, these differences can be overcome if a truly pluralistic approach to planning and implementation of health care service is adopted. The starting point is understanding the culture and structure of the community/region and not treating them as homogeneous.

These issues must be understood within the context of how a health system operates under a political and economic system whose structure and culture is that of capitalism. The basic instrumental mechanism for access and participation in such a system is economic status. The people who have the money have greater access to the system and as I have described, the ones without money would have little or no access if governmental policies did not open the doors for them. The people who fall through the cracks participate little in the system. Thus, a capitalistic system is one of privilege for those with wealth and power. Those communities and individuals that are economically disadvantaged, while generally accepting the dominant ideology, often cannot participate with equal status in the health system.

Poverty, income distribution, and rural underdevelopment are part of a process that can culminate in social marginalization at best and the death of a community at worst (Padfield and Young 1977; Padfield 1980). Community process takes place in a specific political and economic environment, one that is controlled and manipulated by national and international forces. It is in this arena that the health system participates and becomes one of several systems that link the macrolevel systems to the microlevel systems. Often, as in the case of Coberly, the fit is imperfect. The differences and conflicts inherent in the system notwithstanding, a change can occur in the health system which involves a strategy on both structural and symbolic levels for all participants in the system. The changes require a reframing of the structures and symbols. Just as the health system is a projection of the social system itself, changes in one reflect changes in the larger unit— a holographic-type function. Therefore, the structural and ideological changes I suggest naturally involve changes in the larger society, not within a revolutionary context but that of a rational praxis combining action and theory.

These changes are in concert with the projected megatrends for the future that will transform our lives (Naisbitt 1982). While I do not agree with some of Naisbitt's generalizations, he has discussed several directions for change I have delineated in this book. Perhaps the most obvious are the trends from centralization to decentralization and from hierarchies to networking. Other trends are institutional self to self-help and either/or options to multiple options. The movement toward decentralization began over a decade ago and has grown in the past few years in many policy areas. Bottom-up policy is perhaps more visible in state and urban politics and to some extent, industry. A concomitant trend is the move towards networking in decision making, a process whereby people talk to one another and share information, ideas and resources. The "people at the bottom" so to speak, participate and, to some extent, control their destinies through sharing their beliefs, concerns and solutions with the experts and organizers and decision-makers. This approach has been successful in the management of chronic disease in Mississippi (Frate, Johnson and Sharpe 1985).

When these horizontal linkages of people with groups of other people are made, changes become easier and the flow of information within a strictly hierarchal structure is facilitated. Of course, hierarchies will never completely disappear but linkages can be expanded both vertically and horizontally. When people are empowered in a system, they participate more readily in the system. Community involvement is important in providing adequate and appropriate health care and, given the major health problems in this society, individual behavior and support for creating a new health order is imperative. Improving the quality of life for people involves their active participation in all aspects of their lives, including health, as rural peoples move toward wellness. Increased resources from other people/groups allow other individuals/groups to have a choice in their health behavior. Through having a choice, they will have more power to create their own health future.

References

Ahearn, M.
  1979   Health Care in Rural America. U.S. Department of Agriculture, Economics, Statistics and Cooperative Service. Agriculture Information Bulletin No. 428.

Alford, Robert R.
  1975   Health Care Politics: Ideological and Interest Group Barrier to Reform. Chicago: University of Chicago Press.

Alford, Terry W.
  1979   Facility Planning, Design, and Construction of Rural Health Centers. Cambridge: Ballinger Publishing Company.

Altensletter, Christa and James Bjorkman
  1975   Federal Impacts on State Health Policy Lessons from Connecticut and Vermont, p. 61. New Haven: Yale Health Policy Project.

American Medical Association
  1979   Education Programs for the Physician's Assistant. Chicago: American Medical Association.

Anderson, Charles H.
  1970   White Protestant Americans From National Origins to Religious Groups. Englewood Cliffs: Prentice-Hall.

Anderson, Odin W.
  1966   Influence of Social and Economic Research on Public Policy in the Health Field: A Review. Milbank Memorial Fund Quarterly, 44(3):11–48.

Anderson, E.J., L.R. Judd, J.T. May and P.K. New
  1976   The Neighborhood Health Center Program, Its Growth and Problems: An Introduction. L.R. Judd and National Urban Coalition, ed. Washington, D.C.: National Association of Neighborhood Health Centers, Inc.

Apple, Dorrian
  1960   How Laymen Define Illness. Journal of Health and Human Behavior 1(3):219–225.

Beale, C.L.
  1981   Rural and Small Town Population Change, 1970–80. ESS Report 5. Economics and Statistics Service. Washington, D.C.: U.S. Department of Agriculture.

Beale, C.L. and G. Fuguitt
1978   The New Pattern of Nonmetropolitan Population Change. In Social Demography. K.L. Taeuber, L.L. Bumpass and J.A. Sweet, eds. Pp. 157–177. New York: Academic Press.

Beaver, Patricia D.
1986   Rural Community in the Appalachian South. Lexington: University of Kentucky Press.

Begun, James W. and Donald E. Broom
1980   Recent Trends in Physician Supply and Distribution in the South. Chapel Hill: Department of Social and Administrative Medicine, School of Medicine, University of North Carolina.

Bell, B.D.
1975   Mobile Medical Care to the Elderly: An Evaluation. Gerontologist 15(2):100–103.

Berger, P. and T. Luckman
1966   The Social Construction of Reality. New York: Doubleday.

Bergner, Lawrence and Alonzo S. Yerby
1976   Low Income and Barriers: In The Health Gap: Medical Services and Poor, The Use of Health Services. Robert L. Lane, et al., eds. Pp. 27–39. New York: Springer Publishing Co.

Berkanovic, Emil and Leo G. Reeder
1973   Ethnic, Economic, and Social Psychological Factors in the Source of Medical Care. Social Problems 21(2):246–259.

Berkanovic, Emil, Carol Telesky, and Sharon Reeder
1981   Structural and Social Psychological Factors in the Decision to Seek Medical Care for Systems. Medical Care 19(7):693–709.

Bernstein, James D., F.P. Hedge, and C.C. Farran
1979   Rural Health Centers in the United States. The Rural Health Center Development Series. Cambridge: Ballinger Publishing Company.

Bertalanffy, Ludwig
1969   General System Theory. New York: George Braziller, Inc.

Bertelson, David
1967   The Lazy South. New York: Oxford University Press.

Bible, B.L.
1970   Physicians' View of Medical Practice in Non-Metropolitan Communities. Public Health Reports 85:11–17.

Bice, Thomas
1981   Social Science and Health Services Research: Contributions to Public Policy. In Issue in Health Care Policy. J.B. McKinlay, ed. Pp. 1–28. Cambridge: The MIT Press.

Blum, Henrik L.
1976   Expanding Health Care Horizons: From a General Systems Concept of Health to a National Health Policy. Oakland: Third Party Associates, Inc.

Bodenheimer, T.S.
1969   Mobile Units: A Solution to the Rural Health Problem. Medical Care 7(2):144–154.

Bradham, Douglas D. and Deborah A. Freund
1982　A Methodology for Cost Structure Analysis of Subsidized Rural Primary Care Practices. Paper presented at 6th Annual Institute, Jeffersonville, Vermont: American Rural Health Association.

Bridgman, R.F.
1955　The Rural Hospital. Geneva: World Health Organization.

Brooks, Edward F., et al.
1981　New Health Practitioners in Rural Satellite Health Centers: The Past and Future. Journal of Community Health 6(4):246-256.

Brooks, Edward F., P.A. Guild, and J.S. Stein
1981　The Future—If Any—Of New Health Practitioners in Rural Primary Care. Chapel Hill: University of North Carolina, Health Services Research Center.

Brooks, Edward F. and Lisa P. Knelson
1981　Physician's Assistants and Nurse Practitioners: Will They Survive the 1980's. American Journal of Rural Health 7(4):28-33.

Brown, David L.
1978　Racial Disparity and Urbanization, 1960-1970. Rural Sociology 43(3):403-425.

Bruce, Phillip A.
1974　And They All Sang Hallelujah. Knoxville: University of Tennessee Press.

Buntz, Gregory C., T.F. Macaluso and J.A. Azarow.
1978　Federal Influence on State Health Policy. Journal of Health Politics, Policy and Law 3(1):71-86.

Burbank, Fred and Joseph Fraumeni
1972　U.S. Cancer Mortality: Non-White Predominance. Journal of the National Cancer Institute 49:649-652.

Bureau of Census
1978　Population Characteristics. Current Population Reports, Series P-20, No. 324.

Buttel, Frederick H. and William L. Flinn
1975　Sources and Consequences of Agrarian Values in American Society. Rural Sociology 40(2):134-151.

Camaroff, Jean
1983　The Defectiveness of Symbols or the Symbols of Defectiveness? On the Cultural Analysis of Medical Systems. Culture, Medicine and Psychiatry 7:3-20.

Caplan, Nathan
1975　The Use of Social Science by Federal Executives. In Social Research and Public Policies. Gene M. Lyons, ed. Hanover: Public Affairs Center, Dartmouth College.
1979　The Two-Communities Theory and Knowledge Utilization. American Behavioral Scientist 22(3):459-470.

Cappanari, Steven N., et al.
1975　Voodoo in the General Hospital: A Case of Hexing and Regional Enteritis. Journal of the American Medical Association 232(9):938-940.

Carlson, Rick J.
  1975   The End of Medicine. New York: Wiley.
Cash, W.S.
  1941   The Mind of the South. New York: Random House.
Champion, D.M. and D.B. Olsen
  1971   Physician Behavior in Southern Appalachia: Some Recruitment Factors.
          Journal of Health and Social Behavior 12(3):245-252.
Chrisman, Noel J.
  1976   American Patterns of Health-Care-Seeking Behavior. In The American
          Dimension: Cultural Myths and Social Realities. W. Arens and Susan P.
          Montague, eds. Pp. 206-217. New York: Alfred Publishing Co., Inc.
Coleman, Sinclair
  1976   Physician Distribution and Rural Access to Medical Services. The Rand
          Corporation, R-1887-HEW.
Congressional Quarterly
  1977   National Health Issues. Washington, D.C.
  1980   Health Policy: The Legislative Agenda. Washington, D.C.
Coop, James H.
  1976   Diversity of Rural Society and Health Needs. In Rural Health Services:
          Organization Delivery and Use. E.W. Hassinger and L.R. Whiting, eds.
          Pp. 26-37. Ames: Iowa State University Press.
Cooper, J.K. and K. Heald and Michael Samuels
  1967   Affecting the Supply of Rural Physicians. American Journal of Public
          Health 67(8):756-759.
Cordes, S.M.
  1976   Distribution of Physician Manpower. In Rural Health Services: Organization,
          Delivery and Use, E.W. Hassinger and L.R. Whiting, eds. Pp. 56-80.
          North Central Regional Center for Rural Development. Ames: Iowa State
          University Press.
Cornman, John M., Irma T. Elo and Alice S. Hersh
  1981   Health Care in Underserved Rural Areas: A Policy Statement. Washington,
          D.C.: The National Rural Center.
Couto, Richard A.
  1975   Poverty, Politics, and Health Care, An Appalachian Experience, Praeger
          Special Studies in U.S. Economic, Social, and Political Issue. New York:
          Praeger Publishers.
Crichton, Anne
  1981   Health Policy Making: Fundamental Issues in the United States, Canada,
          Great Britain, Australia. Ann Arbor: Health Administration Press.
Cross, H.J. and H.A. Dengerick
  1982   Introduction. In Training Professionals for Rural Mental Health, H.E.
          Dengerick and H.J. Cross, eds. Lincoln: University of Nebraska Press.
D'Andrade, Roy G.
  1984   Cultural Meaning Systems. In Culture Theory: Essays on Mind, Self and
          Emotion, Richard A. Sheder and Robert A. LeVine, eds. Cambridge:
          Cambridge University Press.

Darity, William A.
1977   Health Care for Blacks. Focus 5:4.

Davis, Allison, B.B. Gardner and M.R. Gardner
1941   Deep South: A Social Anthropological Study of Caste and Caste. Chicago: University of Chicago Press.

Davis, Karen
1976   Medicaid Payments and Utilization of Medical Services by the Poor. Inquiry 13(2):122–135.

Davis, Karen and Ray Marshall
1979   New Developments in the Market for Rural Health Care. Research in Health Economics 1:57-110.

Decker, Barry
1977   Federal Strategies and Quality of Local Health Care. In Health Services: The Local Perspective, Arthur Levin, ed. New York: Proceedings of the Academy of Political Science.

De Kadt, Emanuel
1981   Ideology, Social Policy, Health and Health Services: A Field of Complex Interactions. Social Science and Medicine 16:741-752.

Department of Health and Human Services
1986   Prevalence of Selected Chronic Conditions, United States, 1979-81. DHHS Publication No. (PHS) 868-1583.

De Miguel, Jesus M.
1975   A Framework for the Study of National Health Systems. Inquiry 12(2):10-24.

DeWalt, Billie R. and Pertti J. Pelto
1985   Micro and Macro Levels of Analyses in Anthropology. Boulder: Westview Press.

Denham, John W. and C. Glenn Pickard, Jr.
1979   Clinical Roles in Rural Health Centers. The Rural Health Center Development Series. Cambridge: Ballinger Publishing Co.

Department of Health, Education and Welfare
1977   Getting Human Service to People in Rural Areas. Office of Human Development.

Dixon, Marlene and Thomas Bodenheimer
1980   Introduction. In Health Care in Crisis, Marlene Dixon and Thomas Bodenheimer, eds. Pp. i-iv. San Francisco: A Synthesis Publication.

Doherty, J.C.
1979   Public and Private Issues in Nonmetropolitan Government. In Growth and Change in Rural America, G.V. Guguitt and J.C. Doherty, eds. pp. 51-101. Washington, D.C.: Urban Land Institute.

Dollard, John
1937   Class and Caste in a Southern Town. New Haven: Yale University Press.

Douglas, Mary and Aaron Wildavsky
1982   Risk and Culture: An Essay on the Selection of Technical and Environmental Dangers. Berkeley: University of California Press.

Dow, William
    1976   Redemption Denied: An Appalachian Reader, Washington, D.C.: Appalachian Documentation.

Doyal, Lesley
    1981   The Political Economy of Health. Boston: South End Press.

Ducker, Dalia G.
    1977   The Myth of Professional Isolation Among Physicians in Non-Urban Areas. Journal of Medical Education 52(12):991–998.

Easton, David
    1965   A Systems Analysis of Political Life. New York: John Wiley and Sons, Inc.

Eckenfels, Edward J., et al.
    1977   Endemic Hypertension in a Poor Black Rural Community: Can it be Controlled? Journal of Chronic Diseases 30(8):499–518.

Edelman, M.
    1971   Politics as Symbolic Action. New York: Academic Press.
    1977   Political Language: Words that Succeed and Policies that Fail. New York: Academic Press.

Eichhorn, R.L. and T.W. Bice
    1973   Academic Disciplines and Health Services Research. In Health Services Research and R and D in Perspective. E.E. Flook and P.J. Sanayana, eds. Pp. 136–149. Ann Arbor: Health Administration Press.

Elling, Ray H.
    1978   Medical Systems as Changing Systems. Social Science and Medicine 12:107–115.

Elliot, J.E. and J.M. Kearn
    1978   Analysis and Planning for Improved Distribution of Nursing Personnel and Services. Department of Health, Education and Welfare.

Elliot, K.
    1975   The Training of Auxiliaries in Health Care. London: Intermediate Technology Publications, Ltd.

England, J. Lynn, W.E. Gibbons and B.L. Johnson
    1979   The Impact of a Rural Environment on Values. Rural Sociology 44(1):119–136.

Estes, Carol
    1979   The Aging Enterprise. New York: Academic Press.

Etzioni, Amitai
    1977   Health as a Social Prioritiy. In Health Services: The Local Perspective, Arthur Levin, ed. Pp. 8–14. New York: The Academy of Political Science.

Fabrega, Horacio
    1973   Toward a Model of Illness Behavior. Medical Care 11(6):470–484.

Feder, J., J. Hadley, and J. Holahan
    1981   Insuring the Nation's Health. Washington, D.C.: The Urban Institute Press.

Fein, Rashi
  1981 Social and Economic Attitudes. Shaping American Health Policy. In Issues in Health Care Policy. John B. McKinlay, ed. Pp. 29–65. Cambridge: MIT Press.
Feldman, Roger D., M. Deitz and E.F. Brooks
  1978 The Financial Viability of Rural Primary Health Care Centers. American Journal of Public Health 68(10):981–988.
Fitzpatrick, J.P. and R.E. Gould
  1970 Mental Illness Among Puerto Ricans in New York: Cultural Condition of Intercultural Misunderstanding. American Journal of Orthopsychiatry 40:238–239.
Fliegel, Frederick C.
  1976 A Comparative Analysis of the Impact of Industrialism on Traditional Values. Rural Sociology 41(4):431–451.
Ford, Amasa B.
  1978 Epidemiological Priorities As a Baker for Health Policy. Bulletin of the New York Academy of Medicine 54(1):10–22.
Foster, George and Barbara Anderson
  1978 Medical Anthropology. New York: John Wiley and Sons.
Fottler, Myron D.
  1979 Physician Attitudes Toward Physician Extenders: A Comparison of Nurse Practitioners and Physician Assistants. Medical Care 17(5):536–549.
Fox, Renee C.
  1977 The Medicalization and Demedicalization of American Society. Daedalus 106(1):9–22.
Frankenberg, Ronald
  1980 Medical Anthropology and Development: A Theoretical Perspective. Social Science and Medicine 14B:197–207.
Frate, Dennis A., S.A. Johnson and T.R. Sharpe
  1985 Solutions to the Problems of Chronic Disease Management in Rural Settings. The Journal of Rural Health 1:52–59.
Freidson, Eliot
  1970 Profession of Medicine: A Study of the Sociology of Applied Knowledge. New York: Dodd, Mead.
Friedl, John
  1978 Health Care Services and the Appalachian Migrant. Department of Anthropology, Ohio State University, The National Center for Health Services Research, Health Resources Administration, and Department of Health, Education and Welfare.
Fuchs, V.R.
  1975 Who Shall Live? Health Economics and Social Choice. New York: Basic Books.
Gaffney, J.C. and Gerald Glandon, eds.
  1979 Profile and Medical Practice 1979. Chicago: American Medical Association.
Gastil, Raymond D.
  1975 Cultural Regions of the United States. Seattle: University of Washington Press.

Gaustod, Edwin S.
  1975   Religious Demography of the South. In Religion and the Solid South. Samuel S. Hill, Jr., ed. Pp. 143-178. Nashville: Abingdon Press.
Geertz, Clifford
  1973   The Interpretation of Cultures. New York: Basic Books, Inc.
  1975   Ideology as a Cultural System. In Symbols and Society: Essays on Belief Systems in Action, Carole E. Hill, ed. Pp. 11-29. Athens: University of Georgia Press.
Georgia Department of Human Resources
  1981   Predicting Mortality Through Life Passage Stages. Atlanta: Division of Public Health, Department of Human Resources.
  1982   Meeting the Health Needs of Georgians: Objectives for the Future. Atlanta: Division of Public Health, Department of Human Resources.
Gibson, R.M. and C.R. Fisher
  1978   National Health Expenditures: Fiscal Year 1977. Social Security Bulletin 41(7):3-20.
Gil, D.F.
  1970   Violence Against Children; Physical Child Abuse in the United States. Cambridge: Harvard University Press.
Gilford, Dorothy M., et al.
  1981   Rural American in Passage: Statistics for Policy. Washington, D.C.: National Academy Press.
Gillin, John and Emmett J. Murphy
  1951   Notes on Southern Culture Patterns. Social Forces 29(2):422-432.
Goode, Byron J.
  1977   The Heart of What's the Matter: The Semantics of Illness in Iran. Culture, Medicine and Psychiatry 1:25-58.
Goodwin, Alan R.E. and Michael T. Smith
  1979   Rural Mental Health: A Community Perspective. In A Companion to the Life Sciences, Stacey B. Day, ed. New York: Van Nostrand Reinhold Company.
Gouldner, Alvin
  1970   The Coming Crisis in Western Sociology. New York: Basic Books.
Gramsci, Antonio
  1971   Selections from the Prison notebooks. New York: International Publishing Co.
Greenhouse, Carol
  1986   Praying for Justice: Faith, Order and Community in an American Town. Ithaca: Cornell University Press.
Greenlick, M.R., et al.
  1982   Two Decades of Federal Policy for Community Based Care and the Health and Mental Health Split: One State's Move Towards Comprehensiveness. Lexington, Kentucky: Paper presented at the 44th Annual Meeting of the Society for Applied Anthropology.
Guillozet, N.
  1975   Community Mental Health: New Approaches for Rural Areas Using Psychiatric Social Workers. Medical Care 13(1):59-67.

Hackney, Sheldon
1969   Southern Violence. American Historical Review 74(3):906–925.
Hall, Arthur L. and Peter G. Bourne
1973   Indigenous Therapist in a Southern Black Urban Community. Archives of General Psychiatry 28(1):137–142.
Hanft, Ruth S.
1981   Use of Social Science Data for Policy Analysis and Policy-Making. Milbank Memorial Fund Quarterly 59(4):596–613.
Hassinger, Edward W.
1976   Pathways of Rural People to Health Behavior. In Health Services: Organization, Delivery and Use, Edward W. Hassinger and Larry R. Whiting, eds. Pp. 164–171. Ames: Iowa State University Press.
Hassinger, Edward W., Lucille S. Gill and Robert Hageman
1978   A Restudy of Physicians in Twenty Rural Missouri Counties. Columbia: Department of Rural Sociology, University of Missouri.
Hassinger, E.W. and L.R. Whiting, eds.
1976   Rural Health Services: Organization, Delivery and Use. Ames: Iowa State University Press.
Health Services Research Group
1975   Development of the Index of Medical Underservices. Health Services Research 10(2):168–180.
Heaton, H.L. and Allen Dobson
1977   Evaluation of National Health Service Corps and Rural Health Initiative Cities. Washington, D.C.: U.S. Government Report No. HF-625 prepared for OPEL, Contract HSA 240-75-0073, Task Order No. 3.
Heaton, H.L., J.H. Rhodes, L.A. Ritz, et al.
1977   Evaluation of National Health Service Corps and Rural Health Initiative Sites. GOEMET Report No. HFK-625.
Hill, Carole E.
1973   Understanding Rural Culture: Some Methodological and Conceptual Implications. Human Organization 32:217–220.
1976   A Folk Medical Belief System in the Rural South: Some Practical Considerations. Southern Medicine 16:11–17.
1977   Anthropological Studies of the American South. Current Anthropology 18:309–326.
1980   Toward Internationalism: Urban Continuity and Change in a Southern City. In The City in a Hierarchical Perspective, Tom Collins, ed. pp. 53–75. Athens: The University of Georgia Press.
1982   The Meaning of the Religious Campmeeting Experience in the American South. Anthropology and Humanism Quarterly 7:39–44.
1985   Training Manual in Medical Anthropology. Washington, D.C.: Society for Applied Anthropology/American Anthropological Publication No. 18.
1986   Translating Primary Health Care Policies to the Local Level: A Comparison of Rural Communities in the United States and Costa Rica. In Current Health Policy Issues and Alternatives: An Applied Social Science Perspective, Carole E. Hill, ed. Pp. 123–144. Athens: University of Georgia Press.

Hill, Carole E. and Holly Mathews
  1981   Traditional Health Beliefs and Practices Among Southern Rural Blacks:
          A Compliment to Biomedicine. In Social Science Perspectives in the South,
          Merle Black and John Shelton, eds., Pp. 307–322. New York: Gordon and
          Breach, Science Publishers.
Hill, Samuel S., Jr.
  1967   Southern Churches in Crisis. New York: Holt, Rinehart and Winston.
  1972   The South's Two Cultures. In: Religion and the Solid South. Samuel S.
          Hill, Jr., ed., Pp. 24–56. Nashville: Abingdon Press.
Horton, Robin
  1967   African Traditional Thought and Western Science. Africa 37:50–71, 155–
          187.
Howard, Ronald A.
  1971   Dynamic Probabilitic Systems. Semi-Markov and Decision Processes, Vol.
          II. New York: John Wiley and Sons, Inc.
HHS
  1980   Human Services Annual Report, Washington, D.C.: U.S. Department of
          Health and Human Services.
  1984   Health in the United States—1984. Washington: U.S. Department of
          Health and Human Services. CHHS Publication No. (PHS) 85-1232.
Illich, Ivan
  1975   Medical Nemesis: The Exploration of Health. Cuernavaca, Mexico: Centro
          Intercultural de Documentacion.
Isaacs, Gertrude
  1973   The Family Nurse and Primary Health Care in Rural Areas. In: Rural
          and Appalachian Health, Robert L. Nolan and J.L. Schwartz, ed. Pp. 117–
          125. Springfield: Charles C. Thomas.
Ivey, Allen E.
  1981   Counseling and Psychotherapy: Toward a New Perspective. In: Cross
          Cultural Counseling and Psychotherapy, Anthony J. Marsella and Paul B.
          Pedersen, eds. Pp. 279–311. New York: Pergamon Press.
Jagger, F.
  1978   Health Manpower for Rural Areas: Evaluation and Research Issues. Paper
          prepared for the Workshop on Directions in Rural Health Evaluation and
          Research. Annapolis: National Center for Health Service Research.
Janson, Janine, Sandra L. Williams, et al.
  1982   Epidemiological Differences Between Sexual and Physical Child Abuse.
          Journal of American Medical Association 247(24):3344–3348.
Janzen, John M.
  1978   The Comparative Study of Medical Systems as Changing Social Systems.
          Social Science and Medicine 12:121–129.
Jeffery, M.J. and R.E. Reeve
  1978   Community and Mental Health Services in Rural Area: Some Practical
          Issues. Community Mental Health Journal 14(1):54–62.
Johnson, Richard L.
  1978   Rural Hospitals Face Change for a Bright Future. Hospitals 52(2):47–50.

Jones, C.O.
  1976   Why Congress Can't Do Policy Analysis (or Words to that Affect). Policy
         Analysis 2(2):251–264.
Jones, Russell A., et al.
  1981   On the Perceived Meaning of Symptoms. Medical Care 19(7):710–717.
Jones, Yvonne V.
  n.d.   Migration in Montgomery County: A Preliminary Statement. Unpublished
         manuscript, Louisville: University of Louisville.
Jordan, Wilbert C.
  1975   Voodoo Medicine. In Textbook of Black Related Diseases, Richard Allen
         Williams, ed. Pp. 715–738. New York: McGraw-Hill, Inc.
Kane, Robert L.
  1969   Determination of Health Care Priorities and Expectations Among Rural
         Consumers. Health Service Research 4(2):42–151.
  1975   Vector Resolution: A New Tool in Health Planning. Medical Care 13(2):126–
         136.
  1977   Problems in Rural Health Care. In Health Services: The Local Perspective,
         Pp. 136–147. New York: Academy of Political Sciences.
Kane, Robert L., Marilyn Dean and Marian Soloman
  1978   An Overview of Rural Health Care Research. Santa Monica: The Rand
         Corporation, P-6110.
Kane, Robert L. and P.D. McConatha
  1975   The Men in the Middle: A Dilemma of Minority Health Workers. Medical
         Care 13(9):736–743.
Kane, Robert L. and Paul F. Westover
  1976   Rural Health Care Research: Past Accomplishments and Future Challenges.
         In Transcultural Health Care Issues and Conditions, M. Leininger, ed.
         Pp. 123–134. Philadelphia: F.A. Davis Co.
Kane, Robert L. and William M. Wilson
  1977   The New Health Practitioner: The Past as Prologue. Western Journal of
         Medicine 127:254–261.
Kane, Robert L., D.M. Olsen, D. Wright, et al.
  1978   Changes in Utilization Patterns in a National Health Service Corps
         Community. Medical Care 16(10):828–836.
Karpetkin, Rhoda
  1976   A Consumer Perspective on the Professional Responsibility for the Quality
         of Health Care. Bulletin of the New York Academy of Medicine 52(1):44–
         50.
Kennedy, Edward
  1979   Conference Overview. In a National Conference on Health Policy, Planning,
         and Financing the Future of Health Care for Blacks in America. Washington,
         D.C.: Public Health Service Research Proceedings Services, DHEW Pub-
         lication No. 79-3228.
Killian, Lewis
  1970   White Southerners. New York: Random House.

Kilpatrick, James J.
  1969   A Conservative Political Philosophy. In The South: A Central Theme? Monroe L. Billington, ed. Pp. 110–118. New York: Holt, Rinehart and Winston.

Kirk, R.F.H., J.D. Alter, H.E. Browne, et al.
  1971   Family Nurse Practitioners in Eastern Kentucky. Medical Care 9(2):160–168.

Kivett, Vira R. and Jean P. Scott
  1979   The Rural By-Passed Elderly: Perspectives on Status and Needs. Raleigh: North Carolina Agricultural Research Service, Technical Bulletin No. 260.

Kleinman, Joel C. and Ronald W. Wilson
  1977   Are "Medically Underserved Areas" Medically Underserved? Health Services Research 12(2):147–162.

Knobel, Roland J., et al.
  1975   Health Field Concept in Georgia. Journal of the Medical Association of Georgia 64(8):311–313.

Knorr, Karin D.
  1977   Policymakers' Use of Social Science Knowledge: Symbolic or Instrumental? In Using Social Research in Public Policymaking, Carol H. Weiss, ed. Lexington: Lexington Books.

Koos, Earl
  1954   The Health of Regionsville: What the People Thought and Did About It. New York: Columbia University Press.

Lakoff, George and Mark Johnson
  1980   Metaphors We Live By. Chicago: The University of Chicago Press.

La Londe, Mark
  1974   A New Perspective on the Health of Canadians. Ottawa: Information Canada.

Larson, O.F.
  1978   Values and Beliefs of Rural People. In Rural U.S.A.: Persistence and Change. T.R. Ford, ed. Pp. 91–112. Ames: Iowa State University Press.

Lawrence, Robert S., et al.
  1977   Physician Receptivity to Nurse Practitioners: A Study of the Correlates of the Delegation of Clinical Responsibilities. Medical Care 15(4):298–310.

Lee, R.C.
  1979   Identification of Health Manpower: Shortage Area and Development of Criteria for Designation. In Public Health Conference on Records and Statistics, DEH Publication No. (PHS) 79-1214. Washington, D.C.: National Center for Health Statistics.

Lefall, LaSalle D.
  1975   Surgery and Oncology. In: Textbook of Black Related Disease. Richard A. Williams, ed. Pp. 739–760. New York: McGraw-Hill Co.

Lehman, E.W. and A.M. Waters
  1979   Control in Policy Research Institutes: Some Correlates. Policy Analysis 5(2):201–222.

Levin, Arthur, ed.
 1977 Health Services: The Local Perspective. New York: Academy of Political Science.
Liccione, W.J. and S. McAllister
 1974 Attitudes of First-Year Medical Students Toward Rural Practice. Journal of Medical Education 49(5):449–451.
Lieban, Richard
 1974 Medical Anthropology. In Handbook of Social and Cultural Anthropology. John J. Honigmann, ed. Pp. 1031–1072. New York: Rand McNally College Publishing Company.
Lingwood, D.A.
 1979 Producing Usable Research: The First Step in Dissemination. American Behavioral Scientist 22(3):339–362.
Lipscomb, Joseph, et al.
 1979 Health Status Maximization and Manpower Allocation. Research in Health Economics, 1:301–401.
Lowe, George D. and Charles W. Peek
 1974 Location and Lifestyle: The Comparative Explanatory Ability of Urbanism and Rurality. Rural Sociology 39(3):392–420.
Lubchansky, I. and E.G. Gould
 1970 Puerto Ricans Spiritualists View of Mental Illness: The Faith Healer as a Paraprofessional. American Journal of Psychiatry 125:312–321.
Maclachlan, Gretchen
 1974 The Other Twenty Percent: A Statistical Analysis of Poverty in the South. Atlanta: Southern Regional Council, Inc.
Margolis, L.H. and Dale Farran
 1981 Unemployment: The Health Consequences of Children. North Carolina Medical Journal 12:849–850.
Marshall, Ray
 1976 Health Care and Rural Development. Report and Recommendation of the Southern Rural Health Conference. Washington, D.C.: National Rural Center.
Mason, H.R.
 1971 Effectiveness of Student Aid Programs Tied to a Service Commitment. Journal of Medical Education 46(7):575–583.
Mattson, D.E., D.E. Stehr and R.E. Will
 1973 Evaluation of a Program Designed to Produce Rural Physicians. Journal of Medical Education 48(4):323–331.
May, J. Thomas, M.L. Durham and Kon-Ming New
 1980 Structural Conflicts in the Neighborhood Health Center Program: The National and Local Perspectives. Journal of Health Politics, Policy and Law 4(4):581–604.
McCormack, R.C. and C.W. Miller
 1972 The Economic Feasibility of Rural Group Practice. Influence of Non-Physician Practitioners in Primary Care. Medical Care 10(1):73–80.

McDonough, J.R., et al.
 1964   Blood Pressure and Hypertensive Disease Among Negroes and Whites: A Study in Evans County, Georgia. Annals Internal Medicine 61:208–214.
McIntyre, M. and J.P. Madden, eds.
 1977   Directory of State Title V Rural Development Programs. University Park: Penn State University.
McKeown, Thomas J.
 1975   The Determinants of Human Health: Behavior, Environment, and Therapy. In Health Care Teaching and Research, William C. Gibson, ed. Pp. 18–27. Vancouver: Alumni Association and the Faculty of Medicine, University of British Columbia.
McNertney, Walter J. and Donald C. Riedel
 1962   Regionalization and Rural Health Care, An Experiment in Three Communities. Ann Arbor: The University of Michigan.
Mechanic, David
 1962   The Concept of Illness Behavior. Journal of Chronic Disease 15:189–194.
 1966   Response Factors in Illness: The Study of Illness Behavior. Social Psychiatry 1:11–20.
 1972   Human Problems and the Organization of Health Care. In The Nations Health: Some Issues of the Annuals of the Academy of Political and Social Science, Vol. 399. Sylvester E. Berke and Alan W. Heston, eds. Pp. 42–59.
 1981   Some Dilemmas in Health Care Policy. In Issues in Health Care Policy, John B. McKinlay, ed. Pp. 80–94. Cambridge: MIT Press.
Miles, David L. and William A. Rushing
 1976   A Study of Physicians' Assistants in a Rural Setting. Medical Care 14(12):987–995.
Miller, Michael K. and Kelly W. Crader
 1979   Rural-Urban Differences in Two Dimensions of Community Satisfaction. Rural Sociology 44(3):489–504.
Miller, Michael K. and A.E. Luloff
 1981   Who is Rural? A Typological Approach to the Examination of Rurality. Rural Sociology 46(4):608–625.
Mills, C. Wright
 1963   Powers, Politics and People: The Collective Essays of C. Wright Mills. New York: Oxford.
Mintz, Sidney W.
 1977   The So-Called World System: Local Initiative and Local Response. Dialectical Anthropology 2(4):253–270.
Moore, G.T., T.R. Willemain, R. Bonanno, et al.
 1975   Comparison of Television and Telephone for Remote Medical Consultation. New England Journal of Medicine 292(14):729–732.
Moriyama, I.M., et al.
 1971   Cardiovascular Diseases in the U.S. Cambridge: Harvard University Press.
Morrison, P.A. and Wheeler, J.P.
 1976   Rural Renaissance in America?: The Revival of Population Growth in Remote Areas. Population Bulletin 31(3):3–26.

Murphree, Alice H.
1976 Folk Beliefs: Understanding of Health, Illness, and Treatment. In the Health of Rural County: Perspectives and Problems, Richard C. Reynolds, Sam A. Bank and Alice H. Murphree, eds. Pp. 111-123. Gainesville: University Press of Florida.

Murphy, R.L.H. and K.T. Bird
1974 Telediagnosis: A New Community Health Resource. Observations on the Feasibility of Telediagnosis Based on 1,000 Patient Transactions. American Journal of Public Health 64(2):113-119.

Myrdal, Gunnar
1944 American Dilemma: The Negro Problem and Modern Democracy. New York: Harper and Rowe.

Naisbitt, John
1982 Metatrends: Ten New Directions Transforming Our Lives. New York: Warner Books, Inc.

National Center for Health Services Research
1983 Research Activities Report 51.

National Center for Health Statistics
1986 Vital Statistics of the United States, 1981. Vol. 2, Mortality. Part A. Washington, D.C.: U.S. Government Printing Office.

Navarro, Vicente
1975 Social Policy Issues: An Explanation of Composition, Nature and Functions of the Present Health Sector of the United States. Bulletin of the New York Academy of Medicine 51(1):199-234.

Nelson, E.C., A.R. Jacobs and K.G. Johnson
1974 Patients' Acceptance of Physicians on Proper Use of Physician's Assistants. Health Services Reports: 87:467-472.

Neville, Gwen K.
1975 Kinfolds and the Covenant: Ethnic Community Among Southern Presbyterians. In The New Ethnicity, John W. Bennett, ed. Pp. 258-274. 1973 Proceedings of the American Ethnological Society. St. Paul: West Publishing Co.

Newell, Kenneth W., ed.
1975 Health by the People. Geneva: World Health Organization.

Odum, Howard
1936 Southern Regions of the United States. Chapel Hill: University of North Carolina Press.

Ortner, Sherry B.
1984 Theory in Anthropology Since the Sixties. Comparative Studies in Society and History 26:126-166.

Owsley, Frank L.
1949 Plain Folk of the South. Baton Rouge: Louisiana State University Press.

Padfield, Harland
1980 The Expendable Rural Community and the Denial of Powerlessness. In The Dying Community, A. Gallaher and H. Padfield, eds. Pp. 159-185. Albuquerque: University of New Mexico Press.

Padfield, H. and J. Young
   1977   Social Marginalization. In: Rural Poverty and the Policy Crisis, R. Coppedge and C. Davis, eds. Ames: Iowa State University Press.

Parker, Ralph C., Jr., and Andrew A. Sorensen
   1978   The Tides of Rural Physicians: The Ebb and Flow, or Why Physicians Move Out of and Into Small Communities. Medical Care 16(2):157–166.

Parsons, Talcott
   1951   The Social System. Glencoe: The Free Press.

Pattison, E. Mansell and Peter E. Polister
   1980   Community Groups: An Empirical Taxonomy For Evaluation and Intervention. In Evaluation and Action in the Social Environment, R.H. Price and P.E. Politser, eds. Pp. 51–68. New York: Academic Press.

Pearsall, Marian
   1966   Cultures of the American South. Anthropological Quarterly 39(2):128–141.

Pennell, Maryland Y. and Josephine L. Lehman
   1951   Statistical Studies of Heart Disease. Public Health Reports 66(3):57–80.

Perrine, E.L. and D.S. Hall
   1972   Rural Ambulance Service Characteristics and Demands Without Economic Barriers. Appalachia Medicine 4:86–93.

Perry, H.B. and D.W. Fisher
   1980   The Present Status of the Physician Assistant Profession: Results of the Association of Physician Assistant Programs 1978: Arlington: Association of Physician Assistant Programs.

Peterson, John H.
   1975   Black-White Joking Relationships Among Newly-Integrated Faculty. Integrated Education 13(1):33–37.

Phillips, Ulrich B.
   1928   The Central Theme of Southern History. American Historical Review 34(1):30–43.
   1929   Life and Labor in the Old South. Boston: Little, Brown.

Powdermaker, Hortense
   1939   After Freedom: A Cultural Study of the Deep South. New York: Viking Press.

Powles, John
   1974   On the Limitations of Modern Medicine. In: The Challenges of Community Medicine, R. Kane, ed. Pp. 89–112. New York: Springer Publishing Co.

Pozen, Michael W.
   1982   Impact of EMS System Development in Rural Areas. Emergency Medical Services Systems Research Projects. Washington, D.C.: U.S. Department of Health and Human Services.

Quinn, Naomi and Dorothy Holland
   1987   Culture and Cognition. In Cultural Models in Language and Thought. Dorothy Holland and Naomi Quinn, eds. Pp. 1–15. New York: Cambridge University Press.

Quinn, Naomi and Holly Mathews
n.d.   Processes of Disease Diagnosis Among Southern Black Root Doctors. Unpublished Manuscript. Durham: Duke University.

Reed, John
1972   The Ending South. Lexington: Lexington Books.

Reich, Robert V.
1985   Toward a New Public Philosophy. Atlantic Monthly 255(5):68–79.

Rein, Martin
1976   Social Science and Public Policy. New York: Penguin Books.

Rein, Martin and Donald A. Schon
1977   Problem Setting in Policy Research. In Using Social Research in Public Policy Making. Carol H. Weiss, ed. Pp. 235–251. Lexington: Lexington Books.

Report on the National Rural Health Conference
1977   Toward a Health Platform for Rural America. Washington, D.C.: Rural America.

Ricketts, Thomas C., G.H. Defriese and C. Seipp
1979   Some Unintended Consequences of Health Insurance: The Case of Rural-Urban Subsidization. Chapel Hill: Health Services Research Center, University of North Carolina.

Rodin, M., K. Michaelson and G.M. Britan
1978   Systems Theory in Anthropology. Current Anthropology 19(4):747–762.

Roemer, Milton I.
1976   Rural Health Care. St. Louis: C.V. Mosby Company.

Rogers, Perry B.
1979   Some Demographic and Health Characteristics of Region IV, Unpublished manuscript. Atlanta: Public Health Service, Department of Health, Education and Welfare.

Rosen, Beatrice M.
1974   Mental Health and the Poor: Have the Gaps Between the Poor and the Non-poor Narrowed in the Past Decade? Paper presented at the Conference on Social Sciences and Health. American Public Health Association.

Rosenblatt, R.A. and I. Moscovice
1975   Establishing New Rural Family Practices: Some Lessons From a Federal Experience. Family Practice 7:755–763.

Rubin, Morton
1951   Plantation County. Chapel Hill: University of North Carolina Press.

Ruiz, Pedro and John Langrod
1976a   Psychiatry and Folk Healing: A Dichotomy? American Journal of Psychiatry 133(1):95–97.
1976b   The Role of Folk Healers. Community Mental Health Journal 12:392–398.

Rural America
1977   Platform for Rural America. Revised at the Third National Conference on Rural America December 5–7, Washington, D.C.

Rushing, William A. and David L. Miles
  1977   Physicians, Physicians' Assistants, and the Social Characteristics of Patients
          in Southern Appalachia. Medical Care 15(12):1004–1013.
Russell, R.D.
  1970   Black Perceptions of Guidance. The Personnel and Guidance Journal
          48(9):721–728.
Salber, Eva J.
  1979   The Law Advisor as a Community Health Resource. Journal of Health
          Politics, Policy and Law 3:469–477.
  1981   Where Does Primary Care Begin? The Health Facilitator as a Central
          Figure in Primary Care. Israel Journal of Medical Science 17:100–111.
Salger, E.J., S.B. Greene, J.J. Feldman, et al.
  1976   Access to Health Care in the Southern Rural Community. Medical Care
          14(12):971–986.
Sanders, Lyle
  1954   Cultural Differences and Medical Care. New York: Russell Sage Foundation.
Saunders, Elijah and Richard A. Williams
  1975   Hypertension. In Textbook of Black-Related Diseases, Richard A. Williams,
          ed. Pp. 333–358. New York: McGraw-Hill.
Scheffler, R.M., S.G. Yoder, N. Weisfeld, G. Ruby
  1979   Physicians and New Health Practitioners: Issues for the 1980s. Inquiry
          16(3):195–229.
Schmeckebirer, Lawrence F.
  1923   The Public Health Service: Its History, Activities and Organization. Institute
          for Government Research and Service Monographs of the United States,
          No. 10. Baltimore: Johns Hopkins University.
Schoenberger, James et al.
  1974   Hypertension in Holmes County, Mississippi. In Epidemiology and Control
          of Hypertension, Paul Oglesby, ed. Pp. 485–501. New York: Stratton.
Schon, Donald A.
  1979   Generative Metaphor: A Perspective on Problem-Setting in Metaphor and
          Thought. New York: Cambridge University Press.
Sedgwick, Peter
  1973   Illness Mental and Otherwise. The Hasting Center Studies 1:3.
Seham, Max
  1973   Blacks and American Medical Care. Minneapolis: The University Press.
Service, Connie and Eva J. Salber
  1977   Community Health Education: The Law Advisor Approach. Durham:
          Duke University Medical Center.
Sheps, C.G., et al.
  1981   Rural Areas and Personnel Health Services: Current Strategies. American
          Journal of Public Health 71(1):71–82.
Sheps, Cecil G., et al.
  n.d.   An Agenda for Evaluating Rural Primary Care Programs. Chapel Hill:
          Health Service Research Center, University of North Carolina.

Sher, Jonathan
  1983   On the Danger of Thinking That Policy is Reality. Rural America 8:10.
Shimkin, Demitri and Gloria Lowe
  1971   The Black Extended Family: A Basic Rural Institution and a Mechanism of Urban Adaptation.*Unpublished Manuscript. Stanford: University of Illinois and Center for Advanced Study in the Behavioral Sciences.
Sigerist, Henry E.
  1960   The Special Position of the Sick. In On the Sociology of Medicine, dM.E. Roemer, ed. New York: M.D. Publications.
Silverman, Marilyn
  1979   Dependency Mediation, and Class Formation in Rural Guyana. American Ethnologist 6(3):466–490.
Simkins, Francis Butler
  1963   A History of the South. New York: Alfred A. Knopf.
Skaling, Michael M.
  1978   Troubles and Triumphs Mold Small Rural Hospital Education. Hospitals 52(2):55–58.
Snell, John E.
  1967   Hypnosis in the Treatment of "Hexed" Patients. American Journal of Psychiatry 124:311–316.
Snow, Loudell F.
  1978   Sorcerers, Saints, and Charlatans: Black Folk Healer in Urban American Culture. Medicine and Psychiatry 2:69–106.
  1979   Voodoo Illness in the Black Population. In Culture, Cures and Contagion, Norman Klein, ed. Pp. 179–184. Novato: Chandler and Sharp.
Southern Regional Council
  1986   Running Fast and Standing Still: Poverty and Black Economic Growth in Georgia's "Sunbelt Boom." Southern Regional Council Publication.
Stack, Carol
  1977   All Our Kin: Strategies for Survival in a Black Community. New York: Harper and Row.
Starr, Paul
  1984   The Social Transformation of American Medicine. New York: Basic Books.
Suchman, E.A.
  1965   Social Patterns of Illness and Medical Care. Journal of Health and Human Behavior 6(1):2–16.
Sudovar, Steven G. and Patrice Hirsch Feinstein
  1979   National Health Insurance Issues: The Adequacy of Coverage. Roche Laboratories.
Taylor, Mark, W. Dickman, and R. Kane
  1973   Medical Students' Attitudes Toward Rural Practice. Journal of Medical Education 48(10):885–895.
Thacker, S.B., C. Osborne and E.J. Salber
  1978   Health Care Decision Making in Southern County. Journal of Community Health 3(4):347–356.

Thacker, Stephen B., et al.
1979 Primary Care in Durham County. Who Gives Care to Whom? Medical Care 17(1):69–78.

Thomas, C.L. and V. Garrison
1975 A General System View of Community Mental Health. In Progress in Community Mental Health, L. Bellak and H. Barter, eds. Vol. 3, Pp. 265–332. New York: Bruner/Mazel.

Thompson, Edgar T.
1965 The South in Old and New Contexts. In The South in Continuity and Change, John McKinney and Edgar T. Thompson, eds. Pp. 451–480. Durham: Duke University Press.

Tindall, George B.
1974 Beyond the Mainstream: The Ethnic Southerners. Journal of Southern History 40(1):3–18.

Tingling, David C.
1967 Voodoo, Root Work and Medicine. Psychosomatic Medicine 29(5):483–490.

Trouillot, Michel-Rolph
1984 Caribbean Peasantries and World Capitalism: An Approach to Micro-Level Studies. Nieume West-Indische Gids 58:37–59.

Ukeles, J.B.
1977 Policy Analysis: Myth or Reality? Public Administration Review 37(3):223–228.

U.S. Congressional Budget Office
1979 Profile of Health Care Coverage: The Haves and Have Nots. Washington, D.C.: U.S. Government Printing Office.

U.S. Department of Health and Human Services Research
n.d. Who are the Uninsured. National Health Care Expenditures Study, Data Review 1.

U.S. Department of Health, Education and Welfare
1979 Healthy People: The Surgeon General's Report on Health Promotion and Disease Prevention. Washington, D.C.: Public Health Service Publication No. 79-55071.

1980 A Report to the President and Congress on the Status of Health Profession Personnel in the United States. Bureau of Health Manpower. Washington, D.C.: U.S. Government Printing Office.

U.S. Senate, Committee on Appropriations
1974 Report 93:11–46.

Vandiver, Frank E.
1969 The Southerner as Extremist. In The South: A Central Theme? Monroe L. Billington, ed. Pp. 69–76. New York: Holt, Rinehart and Winston.

Vladeck, Bruce C.
1981 Equity, Access, and the Cost of Health Services. Medical Care 19 (Dec. Suppl.):69–79.

Wade, Torlen L. and Edward F. Brooks
1979 Planning and Managing Rural Health Centers. Cambridge: Ballinger Publishing Company.

Wagenfeld, M.O. and J.K. Wagenfeld
  1981   Values, Culture and Delivery of Mental Health Services. In Perspectives on Rural Mental Health, M.O. Wagenfeld, ed. San Francisco: Jossey-Bass Inc.
Waitzkin, Howard
  1978   A Marxist View of Medical Care. Annals of Internal Medicine 89:264–278.
Walker, Mary
  1978   Non-Physician Health Professionals and Rural Health. Yucatan Mexico: Paper presented at the 38th Annual Meeting of the Society for Applied Anthropology in Merida, Yucatan, Mexico.
Wallack, Stanley and Sandra E. Kretz
  1981   Rural Medicine: Obstacles and Solution for Self-Sufficiency. Lexington: Lexington Books.
Warren, David G.
  1979   A Legal Guide for Rural Health Programs. The Rural Health Center Development Series. Cambridge: Ballinger Publishing Company.
Wartow, Nancy J.
  1979   Rural Health at Crossroads: Status and Policy Consideration. Washington, D.C.: Office of Human Development, Department of Health, Education and Welfare.
Weiss, Carol H.
  1977   Introduction. In Using Social Research in Public Policymaking. Carol H. Weiss, ed., pp. 1–20. Lexington: Lexington Books.
  1979   Access to Influence: Some Effects of Policy Sector on the Use of Social Science. American Behavioral Scientist 22(3):437–458.
Weiss, Carol H. and Michael J. Bucuvalas
  1977   The Challenge of Social Research to Decision Making. In Using Social Research in Public Policymaking, Carol H. Weiss, ed. Pp. 213–234. Lexington: Lexington Books.
Weidman, Hazel H.
  1976   In Praise of the Double Bind Inherent in Anthropological Application. In Do Applied Anthropologists Apply Anthropology? Michael Angrosino, ed. Pp. 105–117. Athens: University of Georgia Press.
  1978   Miami Health Ecology Project: A Statement of Ethnicity and Health. Miami: Department of Psychiatry, University of Miami School of Medicine.
Weston, Jerry L.
  1980   Distribution of Nurse Practitioners and Physician Assistants: Implication of Legal Constraints and Reimbursement. Public Health Reports 95(3):253–258.
Wheeler, Raymond
  1976   Summation: Southern Rural Health Conferences. Report and Recommendation of the Southern Rural Health Conference. Washington, D.C.: National Rural Center.
WHO Executive Committee
  1979   Development of Rural Health Teams: Views of a WHO Executive Committee. WHO Chronicle 33(11):407–414.

Williams, Ralph Chester
  1951   The United States Public Health Service. Washington, D.C.: Commissioned
          Officers Association of the United States Public Health Service.
Wintrob, Ronald M.
  1973   The Influence of Others: Witchcraft and Rootwork as Explanations of
          Behavior Disturbances. Journal of Nervous and Mental Disease 156(5):318–
          326.
Withers, Carl
  1946   The Folklore of a Small Town. Transactions of the New York Academy
          of Science 8:234–251.
Wolf, Eric R.
  1982   Europe and the People Without History. Berkeley: University of California
          Press.
Woodward, C. Vann
  1960   The Burden of Southern History. Baton Rouge: Louisiana State University
          Press.
WHO-UNICEF
  1978   Primary Health Care. Geneva: World Health Organization.
Wright, Diana Dryer
  1976   Recent Rural Health Research. Journal of Community Health 2(1):60–72.
Wysong, Jere A.
  1975   The Index of Medical Underservice. Problem in Meaning, Measurement
          and Use. Health Service Research 10(2):127–135.
Zborowski, Mark
  1952   Cultural Comments in Responses to Pain. Journal on Sociological Issues
          8:16–30.
  1969   People in Pain. San Francisco: Jossey-Bass Inc.
Zuiches, James J. and David L. Brown
  1978   The Changing Character of the Nonmetropolitan Population, 1950–1975.
          In Rural U.S.A.: Persistence and Change, Thomas R. Ford, ed. Pp. 55–
          72. Ames, Iowa: Iowa State University Press.

Index